D0209300

WHITE COAT
BLACK HAT

WHITE COAT
BLACK HAT

Adventures on the
Dark Side of Medicine

•

CARL ELLIOTT

BEACON PRESS

BOSTON

BEACON PRESS
25 Beacon Street
Boston, Massachusetts 02108–2892
www.beacon.org

Beacon Press books
are published under the auspices of
the Unitarian Universalist Association of Congregations.

13   12   11   10   8   7   6   5   4   3   2   1

This book is printed on acid-free paper that meets the uncoated paper
ANSI/NISO specifications for permanence as revised in 1992.

Text design and composition by Yvonne Tsang
at Wilsted & Taylor Publishing Services

A version of the chapter "The Guinea Pigs" appeared in the *New Yorker*
under the title "Guinea-Pigging"; a version of the chapter "The Detail Men"
appeared in the *Atlantic Monthly* under the title "The Drug Pushers."

Library of Congress Cataloging-in-Publication Data

Elliott, Carl, 1961–
White coat, black hat: Adventures on the Dark Side
of Medicine. / Carl Elliott.
p. ; cm.
Includes bibliographical references and index.
ISBN 978-0-8070-6142-8 (hardcover : alk. paper)
1. Medical ethics—United States. 2. Pharmaceutical industry—
United States. 3. Medicine—United States. I. Title.
[DNLM: 1. Drug Industry—ethics. 2. Conflict of Interest.
3. Drug Evaluation—ethics. 4. Ethics, Medical. 5. Professional
Misconduct. QV 736 E46w 2010]

R724.E385 2010
174.2′951—dc22
2010006119

In memory of Cliff Geertz

CONTENTS

INTRODUCTION

IN THE SUMMER OF 1989 my younger brother, Hal, began his residency in psychiatry. One of his fellow residents was a recent Harvard graduate, whom I will call Len Shoemaker, who had come to the program with the reputation of an academic star. Shoemaker did not have merely a Harvard medical degree. He also had a PhD in neuroscience. He had impressed faculty members while doing a clinical elective as a visiting medical student the year before, and during that time he became engaged to a psychiatry resident. The two married shortly afterward and began looking for a way to continue their psychiatry training in the same city.

Hal did not warm to Shoemaker. Not that he and Shoemaker ever had a direct confrontation, or even exchanged harsh words. But Shoemaker had an obsequious manner that made Hal uneasy. "He reminded me of Eddie Haskell on *Leave It to Beaver*," Hal says. "You know, 'That's a very nice dress you're wearing, Mrs. Cleaver.'" It was not just that Shoemaker tried to ingratiate himself with attending physicians. This is a time-honored medical tradition. But Shoemaker also tried to ingratiate himself with his fellow residents. Hal says, "I always asked myself: why would he be sucking up to me?"

Shoemaker's manner would have been easy to overlook if he had pulled his weight in the hospital. But he often tried to weasel his way out of taking call, and he would even pretend to be sick in order to avoid working up patients. During the first year of the residency, a rumor began to circulate that Shoemaker was having an affair with another psychiatry resident. Later, a similar rumor emerged about an affair with a hospital attorney. The residents began to wonder: *What is he thinking?*

Does his wife know what is going on? Yet the faculty members had no serious complaints about the quality of Shoemaker's work. His evaluations were fine, and Shoemaker finished the first year of his residency without a major hitch.

That soon changed. First-year residents practice medicine with a provisional license, and as Shoemaker entered his second year of residency training, he applied to the state Board of Medical Examiners for a full medical license. Standard procedure required the board to verify Shoemaker's credentials with the American Medical Association. Surprisingly, the AMA replied that it had no file on Shoemaker. The board then contacted Harvard University. Harvard said it had no record of Shoemaker either. When Shoemaker was summoned by the residency director to explain the discrepancy, he said, "I'll need to talk to my attorney." Then he disappeared. Nobody in the Department of Psychiatry has seen him since that day.

It turned out that Shoemaker was a fraud. He had never graduated from medical school. He didn't have a PhD in neuroscience. It is possible that he never even graduated from college. Because Shoemaker was admitted to the residency program outside the regular channels, no one had ever formally checked his credentials. Not even his wife knew who he really was. He had forged everything he needed to get into the program, including a letter from the associate dean of Harvard Medical School. Some rumors suggested that he may have worked as a technician in a hospital in Texas, where he could have picked up some technical skills and learned hospital jargon, but as far as anyone could officially determine, Shoemaker had practiced psychiatry as a resident for fourteen months without any formal medical training at all.

The most striking thing about Shoemaker's fraud is how completely he deceived everyone at the university, in spite of his obvious flaws. When Shoemaker applied for the residency, he was interviewed by four different faculty members, each of whom gave him a rating of "outstanding." He did clinical rotations not just in psychiatry but in internal medicine and neurology, and he fooled those attending physicians as well. "There were times when I thought, Man, for someone with a PhD from Harvard, this guy just sucks," says Hal. But he never suspected that Shoemaker might be a fraud. Nor, apparently, did any of the other residents. "What we thought was that he was a narcissistic sociopath," Hal says. "We never thought that he wasn't a doctor." Then he adds, "Actually, being a narcissistic sociopath is kind of a prerequisite for medical school. Maybe that's why he was so convincing."

Over the years Hal and I have spent many hours talking about the Shoemaker story. But while I still marvel at Shoemaker's ingenuity, I am no longer shocked by his fakery. I'm not sure when my perspective changed. It may have been when I met a biologist who writes fake-scientific articles for the drug industry. It could have been when a friend confided that he used to produce fake television news stories promoting new drugs, or when a physician-researcher in Alabama was sent to federal prison for faking data in a clinical trial of the antibiotic Ketek. But the real turning point probably occurred when I came across a community of professional research subjects who fake their medical histories to get into high-paying clinical studies, then fake painful side effects when they want to get out. Fake science, fake news, fake researchers, fake subjects: sometimes it seems to me that Len Shoemaker is emblematic of what American medicine has become.

Not all of medicine, of course. There are still plenty of honest doctors out there. But honesty is getting harder all the time. Without actually intending it, we have constructed a medical system in which deception is often not just tolerated but rewarded. A series of social and legislative changes have transformed medicine into a business, yet because of medicine's history as a self-regulating profession, no one is really policing it. On the surface, our medical system looks very similar to the way it looked twenty-five years ago. Dig deeper, though, and you can see the same patterns of misconduct emerging again and again. If Len Shoemaker were to resurface today, it would not surprise me to learn that he had become a successful pharmaceutical executive.

It is tempting to blame these problems on pharma, especially after so many high-profile revelations about industry misconduct. And it is true that this misconduct has been integrated into an extraordinarily successful business model. For years the pharmaceutical industry has been among the most profitable industries in the world, even by the exceptionally high standards of, say, the mining or oil industry. For much of the 1990s, pharma was the world's single most profitable business, as measured by *Fortune* magazine, and even in 2009, after several years of litigation, layoffs, and expiring patents, it ranked third.[1] Often overlooked, however, is the extent to which the pharmaceutical industry has changed the practice of medicine itself, especially in academic health centers. It is not simply that academic physicians attend Continuing Medical Education courses underwritten by the pharmaceutical industry, sign journal articles written by industry-appointed ghostwriters, conduct clinical trials sponsored by the drug industry, and eat lunch courtesy of industry drug reps. It is that universities themselves must compete in a marketplace dominated by the industry and its commercial spin-offs. If more academics think like businesspeople now, it is partly because the world in which drugs are tested, developed, and marketed is so completely ruled by business.

This is not entirely new. For as long as there has been a pharmaceutical industry, there have been efforts by the pharmaceutical industry to befriend doctors, often with payments and gifts. My father is a family doctor in South Carolina, and my brothers and I grew up in the 1970s tossing Merck Frisbees and playing with Pfizer Nerf balls. When I finished medical school, I was presented with a doctor's bag paid for by Eli Lilly. Over the years I have carried Zithromax umbrellas, drunk from Inderal coffee cups, and eaten more industry-sponsored pizzas than I can count. After my second year of medical school I spent a summer working in the medical department of SmithKline Beecham in Munich. In retrospect, the work I did for them was pretty worthless, but at the time, the job seemed like a gift. Which, I suppose, it was.

In the 1980s, when I was studying philosophy at Glasgow University in Scotland, I became involved with the Glasgow Medical Group, a student organization that sponsored lectures and debates in medical ethics. The group was run on a shoestring budget. Guest lecturers donated their time to the group, and we often entertained them with potluck dinners at student flats. The Edinburgh Medical Group, in contrast, a similar but better-funded organization fifty miles to the east, was rumored to accept donations from the pharmaceutical industry. Inevitably, the question was raised: Should we do the same?

I always argued yes. Part of it was sheer hardheadedness. I was the only American and I felt defensive about American values, surrounded as I was by Glaswegian socialists. But I also genuinely believed my own arguments. I honestly didn't think that industry funding would compromise the group in any way. The funding would make no difference to the content of the lectures, and I was convinced it would make no difference to the attitudes of individual members of the group. Take the money, I argued; just do and say what you want. Looking back, though, I can't help but wonder if the reason I was so convinced was that I had already taken so much industry charity myself.

My feelings about the drug industry began to turn in the 1990s. This may have been because my jobs took me further away from my medical-school indoctrination, or it may have been because I was living in New Zealand and then Canada, where citizens are much less comfortable with free-market thinking. But this was also a time when the drug industry and its corporate partners became much more influential. When I moved back to the United States in 1997, television stations had started running ads for prescription drugs in their prime-time evening lineups. Strange new pharma-related companies had emerged, often with unfamiliar acronyms (CROs, SMOs, MECCs, NIRBs). The drug industry had expanded its armies of drug reps, who were much younger and better-looking than I remembered, and one of them always seemed to be standing next to me in the hospital elevator carrying chocolate doughnuts and smiling. As the commercial aims of the industry became more direct, any illusion that the business was engaged in a humanitarian enterprise began to fall away. The pharma doughnuts began to sit uneasily in my stomach.

For the first time, I started to think about the people carrying the doughnuts. I had never paid much attention to drug reps before, much less to public relations specialists, thought leaders, or ghostwriters. The better I got to know the reps, the more closely they seemed to resemble con men, a genre of criminal for which I have a certain grudging admiration. There is something intriguing about a well-executed scam. To listen to a first-rate drug rep explain how he games the medical system is a little like listening to a crooked carnie at the state fair explain how he fixes the contests so that the house always wins. It is disconcerting to find out the system is rigged, but once the initial shock wears off, your natural question is: How did they do it?

The answer is often deceptively simple. A well-played confidence trick takes advantage of certain predictable characteristics of human psychology—the susceptibility to flattery, the deference to authority and status, the willingness of the eye to see what it wants to see and ignore the rest. Like a good scam artist, a good drug rep or PR expert figures out what a mark wants to believe and then gently helps him believe it. The most interesting kinds of scams reveal larger insights about the way we live now—the things we desire, the sources of our fears, the nature of our aspirations. While I can't exactly endorse the ethics of the scam, I can't help but admire the cunning required to carry it off.

Of course, some of the best stories come not from the scam artists themselves but from the people who have been scammed. Conventional wisdom says that people are lured into confidence tricks by greed, and sometimes this is true. In medicine, however, the scams often take advantage of a person's good intentions. The ingenuity of the scam comes from the way it plays on a well-intentioned person's desire to help the sick and disabled, or enlist others in the cause of justice, or bring health care to the poor. My best informants have enough detachment to see what made them so vulnerable to deception. And, of course, there is also something enormously appealing about people who are willing to talk openly about their personal humiliation.

Like an exam cheat at a school with an honor code or a burglar in a town where nobody locks the door, a scam artist will find his job easier in a place of honesty and trust. It also helps if his marks are extraordinarily self-confident, convinced of their own intelligence and moral integrity. The best mark is often a person to whom the possibility of a con never occurs, simply because he thinks he is too smart to be tricked. Medical practice is a little like this. Many doctors know nothing about advertising, salesmanship, or public relations. They believe these are jobs for people who could not get into medical school. This is probably why doctors are so easily fooled.

In some ways, the changes in medicine over the past two decades resemble the changes of the Internet. In the late 1980s and early '90s, the Internet was used mainly in government offices and universities. Back in those days, e-mail was a great but little-known perk of academic life. The main challenge was trying to convince other people to use it. Nobody worried too much about things like fraud or deception, and there was no real need to. University life was based on trust and openness, at least by the standards of business, and while people didn't exactly trust what they read online, they did not spend much time fretting over being cheated.

Within a decade, however, everything changed. By the early 2000s, the Internet had been transformed into a vast commercial venture. This was the era of Amazon.com, eBay, and PayPal. Everyone began shopping online, banking online, and dating online. Commerce made the Internet more interesting, but also darker and more dangerous. The early spirit of openness had created a window of vulnerability, and many strange people were trying to crawl through it. You had to watch the window constantly for spammers and frauds and spies. Today, anyone with an e-mail address has to be vigilant about identity thieves, Viagra peddlers, and rich Nigerian widows.

Something similar has happened with American health care. Doctors used to be more powerful than health-care corporations; medicine was once seen as a profession, not a business; and medical research was housed largely in universities. The ethos of medicine simply assumed a kind of openness. The scientific community trusted that researchers

were behaving honestly. Physicians published studies for free in journals, and even paid publishers for reprints. Today, of course, things are
very different. The financial stakes in medical enterprises are enormous;
the center of drug research has moved to the private sector; even medical education has become big business. Like the Internet, medicine has
been transformed by commerce. And just as the ethos of trust opened a
window for deception on the Internet, so it opened a window for deception in medicine.

But medicine and the Internet differ dramatically in one important
way: The Internet has adapted to the commercial era. It does not operate
on trust anymore. Everyone protects his or her computer with firewalls,
virus scanners, anti-spyware programs, and spam detectors. The same is
not true for medicine. Health care may be a business now, but it still operates by the old rules. Medical journals still trust authors; patients still
trust doctors; researchers trust subjects; and subjects trust researchers.
Nobody wants to admit that the world has changed. Nobody is willing to
concede that trust may no longer be warranted.

Of course, trust and honesty are a lot less entertaining than fraud,
bribery, and misdirection. I do not claim to offer a balanced picture of
contemporary American medicine. My interest is in how medicine has
gone wrong, not in what there is to admire. Nor have I tried to draw a
comprehensive chart of American health care. Our health-care system
has grown up over years, accidentally and unplanned, like the streets
of an old city. I am less concerned with mapping out that city than in
exploring what it is like to work those streets.

Those streets are also changing quickly. Anyone who has tried to
document the relationship between medicine and industry will know
how difficult it is to keep up with all the shifts and turnarounds: the
marketing scandals, clinical-trial disasters, government investigations,
and whistle-blower lawsuits, each of which seems to prompt a series of
institutional responses—a new professional ethics code, a different set
of Pharmaceutical Research and Manufacturers of America (PhRMA)
guidelines, a revised FDA guidance. Eventually I decided that it was less
important to document each legal action and bureaucratic reaction than
it was to understand the roots and scope of the problem.

As this book goes to press, signs are emerging that the relationship
between medicine and industry may be on the verge of more significant change. Pfizer has settled the largest health-care fraud lawsuit in
American history. Many universities have announced new conflict-of-
interest policies. The Senate Finance Committee continues to investi-

gate academic physicians who consult and speak for industry. Sunshine laws are being proposed and, in some cases, put into place, illuminating the hidden financial ties between industry and its marketing vehicles. But as history shows, the relationship between American medicine and industry has never been completely severed. I doubt that their financial ties will disappear anytime soon.

WHITE COAT
BLACK HAT

CHAPTER ONE

The Guinea Pigs

O N SEPTEMBER 11, 2001, James Rockwell was camped out in a clinical-research unit on the eleventh floor of a Philadelphia hospital where he had enrolled as a subject in a high-paying drug study. As a rule, studies that involve invasive medical procedures are more lucrative—the more uncomfortable, the better the pay—and in this study, subjects had a fiber-optic tube inserted in their mouths and down their esophaguses so that researchers could examine their gastro-intestinal tracts.

Rockwell had enrolled in many previous studies at corporate sites, places like Wyeth and GlaxoSmithKline. But the atmosphere there felt professional, bureaucratic, and cold. This unit was in a university hospital, not a corporate lab, and the staff had a casual attitude toward regulations and procedures. "The Animal House of research units" is what Rockwell calls it. "I'm standing in the hallway juggling," he says. "I'm up at five in the morning watching movies." Although study guidelines called for stringent dietary restrictions, the subjects got so hungry that one of them picked the lock on the food closet. "We got giant boxes of cookies and ran into the lounge and put them in the couch," Rockwell says. "This one guy was putting them in the ceiling tiles." Rockwell has little confidence in the data that the study produced. "The most integral part of the study was the diet restriction," he says, "and we were just gorging ourselves at two a.m. on Cheez Doodles."

On the morning of September 11, nearly a month into the five-week study, the subjects gathered around a television and watched the news of the terrorist attacks through a drug-induced haze. "We were all high on Versed after getting endoscopies," Rockwell says. He and the other subjects began to wonder if they should go home. But a mass departure would have ruined the study. "The doctors were like 'No, no!'" Rockwell recalls. "'No one's going home, everything's fine!'" Rockwell stayed until the end of the study and was paid seventy-five hundred dollars. He used the money to make a down payment on a house.

Rockwell is a wiry thirty-year-old massage-therapy student with a pierced nose; he seems to bounce in his seat as he speaks, radiating enthusiasm. Over the years, he has enrolled in more than twenty studies for money, he estimates. The Philadelphia area offers plenty of opportunities for aspiring human subjects. It is home to four medical schools and is part of a drug-industry corridor that stretches from there into New Jersey. Bristol-Myers Squibb regularly sends a van to pick up volunteers at the Trenton train station.

Today, fees as high as the one that Rockwell received in 2001 aren't unusual. The best-paying studies are longer, inpatient trials, where subjects are often required to check into a research facility for days or even weeks at a time so that their diets can be controlled, their blood and urine tested regularly, and their medical status carefully monitored. Occasionally, they also undergo invasive procedures, like bronchoscopies or biopsies, or suffer through something else unpleasant, such as being deprived of sleep, wearing a rectal probe, or having allergens sprayed in their faces. Because such studies require a fair amount of time in a research unit, the usual subjects are people who need money and have a lot of time to spare: the unemployed, college students, contract workers, ex-cons, or young people living on the margins who have decided that testing drugs is better than punching a clock with the wage slaves. In some cities, like Philadelphia and Austin, the drug-testing economy has produced a community of semiprofessional research subjects who enroll in one study after another. Some of them do nothing else. For them, guinea-pigging, as they call it, has become a job. Many of them say that they know people who have been traveling around the country doing studies for fifteen years or longer. "It's crazy and it's sad," one drug-trial veteran told me. "For me, this is not a life. But it is a life for a lot of these people."

•   •   •

Most drug studies used to take place in medical schools and teaching hospitals. Pharmaceutical companies developed the drugs, but they contracted with academic physicians to carry out the clinical testing. According to the *New England Journal of Medicine*, as recently as 1991,

80 percent of industry-sponsored trials were conducted in academic health centers. Academic health centers had a lot to offer pharmaceutical companies: researchers who could design the trials, publications in reputable journals that could help market the products, and a pool of potential subjects on whom the drugs could be tested. But in the past decade or so, the pharmaceutical industry has been testing more drugs, the trials have grown more complex, and the financial pressure to bring drugs to market swiftly has intensified. Impatient with the slow pace of academic bureaucracies, pharmaceutical companies have moved trials to the private sector, which is where more than 70 percent of them were conducted in 2004.[1]

This has spurred the growth of businesses that specialize in various parts of the commercial-research enterprise. The largest of the new businesses are called contract research organizations (CROs) and include Quintiles, Covance, Parexel, and PPD (Pharmaceutical Product Development), a company that has operations in thirty countries, including India, Israel, and South Africa. These firms are hired to shepherd a product through every aspect of its development, from subject recruitment and testing through FDA approval. Speed is critical: a patent lasts twenty years, and a drug company's aim is to get the drug on the shelves as early in the life of the patent as possible. In 2000, when the Office of Inspector General of the Department of Health and Human Services asked one researcher what sponsors were looking for, he replied, "Number one—rapid enrollment. Number two—rapid enrollment. Number three—rapid enrollment."[2] The result has been a broadening of the range of subjects who are used and an increase in the rates of pay they receive.

Most professional guinea pigs are involved in Phase I clinical trials, in which the safety of a potential drug is tested, typically by giving it to healthy subjects and studying any side effects that it produces. (Phase II trials aim to determine dosing requirements and demonstrate therapeutic efficacy; Phase III trials are on a larger scale and usually compare a new drug's results with those of standard treatments.) The better trial sites offer such amenities as video games, pool tables, and wireless Internet access. If all goes well, a guinea pig can get paid to spend a week watching *The Lord of the Rings* and playing Halo with his friends in exchange for wearing a hep-lock catheter in one arm and eating institutional food. Nathaniel Miller, a Philadelphia drug-trial veteran who started doing studies in order to fund his political activism, was once paid fifteen hundred dollars in exchange for three days and two endoscopies at Temple University, where he was given a private room with a television. "It was like a hotel," he says, "except that twice they came in and stuck a tube down my nose."

The shift to the market has created a new dynamic. The relationship between testers and test subjects has become, more nakedly than ever, a business transaction. Guinea pigs are the first to admit this. "Nobody's doing this out of the goodness of their heart," Miller says. Unlike subjects in later-stage clinical trials, who are usually sick and might enroll in a study to gain access to a new drug, people in healthy-volunteer studies cannot expect any therapeutic benefit to balance the risks they take. As guinea pigs see it, their reason for taking the drugs is no different from that of the clinical investigators who administer them and who are compensated handsomely for their efforts. This raises an ethical question: what happens when both parties involved in a drug trial see the enterprise primarily as a way of making money?

· · ·

In May of 2006, Miami-Dade County ordered the demolition of a former Holiday Inn, citing various fire and safety violations. It had been the largest drug-testing site in North America, with six hundred and seventy-five beds. The operation had closed down earlier that year, shortly after the financial magazine *Bloomberg Markets* reported that the building's owner, SFBC International, was paying undocumented immigrants to participate in drug trials under ethically dubious conditions.[3] The medical director of the clinic had gotten her degree from a school in the Caribbean and was not licensed to practice. Some of the studies had been approved by a commercial ethical review board owned by the wife of an SFBC vice president. (The company, which has since changed its name to PharmaNet Development Group, says that it required subjects to provide proof of their legal status, and that the practice of medicine wasn't part of the medical director's duties. In August 2007 the company paid $28.5 million to settle a class-action lawsuit.[4])

"It was a human-subjects bazaar," says Kenneth Goodman, a bioethicist at the University of Miami who visited the site. The motel was in a downtrodden neighborhood; according to later reports, paint was peeling from the walls, and there were seven or eight subjects in a room. Goodman says that the waiting area was filled with potential subjects, mainly African American and Hispanic; administrative staff members worked behind a window, like gas-station attendants, passing documents through a hole in the glass.

4

The SFBC scandal was not the first of its kind. In 1996, the *Wall Street Journal* reported that at its testing site in Indianapolis, Eli Lilly and Company was using homeless alcoholics from a local shelter to test experimental drugs at budget rates. (Lilly's executive director of clinical pharmacology told the *Journal* that the homeless people were driven by "altruism" and that they enrolled in trials because they "want to help society." The company says that it now requires subjects to provide proof of residence.) The Lilly clinic, the *Journal* reported, had developed such a reputation for admitting the down-and-out that subjects traveled to Indianapolis from all over the country to participate in studies.[5]

How did the largest clinical-trial unit on the continent recruit undocumented immigrants to a dilapidated motel for ten years without anyone's noticing? Part of the answer has to do with our system of oversight. Before the 1970s, medical research was poorly regulated; many Phase I subjects were prisoners. Reforms were instituted after congressional investigations into abuses like the four-decade-long Tuskegee syphilis studies, in which researchers observed, instead of treating, syphilis infections in African American men. For the past three decades, institutional review boards, or IRBs, have been the primary mechanism for protecting subjects in drug trials. FDA regulations require that any study in support of a new drug be approved by an IRB. Until recently, IRBs were based in universities and teaching hospitals and were made up primarily of faculty members who volunteered to review the research studies being conducted in their own institutions. Now that most drug studies take place outside academic settings, research sponsors can submit their proposed studies to for-profit IRBs, which will review the ethics of a study in exchange for a fee. These boards are subject to the same financial pressures faced by virtually everyone in the business. They compete for clients by promising a fast review. And if one for-profit IRB concludes that a study is unethical, the sponsor can simply take it to another.[6]

Moreover, because IRBs scrutinize studies on paper only, they are seldom in a position to comment on conditions at a study site. Most of the standards that SFBC violated in Miami, for example, would not be evaluated in an ordinary off-site ethics review. IRBs ask questions like "Have the subjects been adequately informed of what the study involves?" They do not generally ask if the sponsors are recruiting undocumented immigrants or if the study site poses a fire hazard. At some trial sites, guinea pigs are housed under conditions that would drive away anyone with better options. Guinea pigs told me about sites that skimp on meals and hot water or that require subjects to bring their own towels and blankets. A few sites have a reputation for recruiting subjects who are threatening or dangerous but who work cheap.

Few people realize how little oversight the federal government provides for the protection of subjects in privately sponsored studies. The Office for Human Research Protections, in the Department of Health and Human Services, has jurisdiction only over research funded by the department. The FDA oversees drug safety, but, according to a 2007 HHS report, it conducts "more inspections that verify clinical trial data than inspections that focus on human-subject protections."[7] In 2005, FDA inspectors were finally given a code number for reporting "failure to protect the rights, safety, and welfare of subjects," and an agency spokesman says that they planned to make more human-subject-safety inspections in the future, but as of early 2008 they had cited only one investigator for a violation. (A psychiatrist had held a research subject in his Oklahoma research facility against her will for four days after she tried to drop out of a drug trial. The psychiatrist had also been disciplined by the state licensing board for giving herpes to two of his patients.[8]) In any case, the FDA inspects only about 1 percent of clinical trials.[9]

The guinea-pig pro has a delicate relationship with trial recruiters. Technically speaking, recruiters are supposed to frown on the practice of serial guinea-pigging. It is not clear what sort of data is generated by trials on people who have recently been taking many other drugs. Nor is it clear what toll these experimental drugs are taking on the long-term health of the guinea pigs themselves. For these reasons, most sites require that guinea pigs wait at least a month after one trial has ended before enrolling in another one. In practice, however, that requirement is sometimes handled with a wink and a nod. If a guinea pig behaves in a study, he may find himself recruited for a new one before he even leaves the trial site.

Yet because their motivation for doing studies is purely financial, guinea pigs have a concrete incentive to lie about their medical history in order to qualify. "If you don't lie then you're talking yourself out of a job," one guinea pig told me. Guinea pigs learn never to admit that they have been sick, that they have used illicit drugs, or that they have recently been in another study. However, once guinea pigs are accepted into a study, they are given financial incentives to stay in. Many sponsors penalize guinea pigs for missing follow-up appointments, and some back-load the pay scale so that guinea pigs have to stay in a study until the end in order to get most of their money. The only way for a subject to get out of a study without being penalized is to experience side effects so severe that the sponsors decide the guinea pig must be dropped.

James Rockwell told me of a time when he enrolled in a thirty-day outpatient study of a drug for Alzheimer's disease that required him to get dosed every morning before he went to work; he painted houses, which involved standing on high ladders. At one point during the study Rockwell decided to leave town to participate in a political demonstration. But this would have meant forfeiting part of his pay. "I decided to fake a story about fainting on the job," he says, which meant he'd be dropped from the study but would still get paid. The Merck doctors tried to persuade him to drop out of the study voluntarily, but Rockwell stood his ground. When he was eventually dropped, it was with full compensation.

Most guinea pigs rely on their wits—or on word of mouth from other subjects—to determine which studies are safe. Some avoid particular kinds of studies, such as trials for heart drugs or psychiatric drugs. Others have developed relationships with certain recruiters whom they trust to tell them which studies to avoid. In general, guinea pigs figure that sponsors have a financial incentive to keep them healthy. "The companies don't give two shits about me or my personal well-being," Nathaniel Miller says. "But it's not in their interest for anything to go wrong." That's true, but companies also have an interest in things going well as cheaply as possible, and this can lead to hazardous trade-offs.

The most notorious recent disaster for healthy volunteers took place in March 2006 at a testing site run by Parexel at Northwick Park Hospital, outside London; subjects were offered two thousand pounds to enroll in a Phase I trial of a monoclonal antibody, a prospective treatment for rheumatoid arthritis and multiple sclerosis. Six of the volunteers had to be rushed to a nearby intensive care unit after suffering life-threatening reactions—severe inflammation, organ failure. They were hospitalized for weeks, and one subject's fingers and toes were amputated. All the subjects have reportedly been left with long-term disabilities.[10]

The Northwick Park episode was not an isolated incident. Traci Johnson, a previously healthy nineteen-year-old student, committed suicide in a safety study of Eli Lilly's antidepressant Cymbalta in January of 2004.[11] (Lilly denies that its product was to blame.) I spoke to an Iraqi living in Canada who began doing trials when he immigrated. He was living in a hostel and needed money to buy a car. A friend told him, "This thing is like fast cash." When he enrolled in an immunosuppressant trial at a Montreal-based subsidiary of SFBC, he found himself in a bed next to a subject who was coughing up blood. Despite his complaints, he was not moved to a different bed for nine days. He and eight other subjects later tested positive for tuberculosis.[12]

•   •   •

A decade ago, shortly after I began teaching bioethics and philosophy at the University of Minnesota, I got a phone call from a psychiatrist named Faruk Abuzzahab. He wanted to know if he could sit in on an ethics class that I was teaching. There had been some trouble in a research study that he had conducted, it seemed, and the state licensing board had ordered him to take a class in medical ethics.

Despite some misgivings about my class being used as an instrument of punishment, I agreed. He seemed affable enough on the phone, explaining that he had been a faculty member at the university before going into private practice and had once chaired the Minnesota Psychiatric Society's ethics committee.

I did not give much more thought to Abuzzahab until several years later, when a for-profit testing site called Prism Research opened in St. Paul. Prism was advertising for healthy subjects in a local alternative weekly. I discovered, on the company's Web site, that Abuzzahab was one of its researchers. A few more clicks revealed that he was also conducting studies at his private practice, Clinical Psychopharmacology Consultants. I began to wonder what, exactly, the incident was that had brought him to my class.

As it turned out, the disciplinary action was a response to the injuries or deaths of forty-six patients under Abuzzahab's supervision. Seventeen of them had been research subjects in studies that he was conducting. These were not healthy-volunteer studies. According to the board, Abuzzahab had "enrolled psychiatrically disturbed and vulnerable patients into investigational drug studies without ensuring that they met eligibility criteria to be in the study and then kept them in the study after their conditions deteriorated." The board had judged Abuzzahab a danger to the public and suspended his license, citing "a reckless, if not willful, disregard of the patients' welfare."

One case, which was reported in the *Boston Globe*, concerned a forty-one-year-old woman named Susan Endersbe, who had struggled for years with schizophrenia and suicidal thoughts. She had been doing well on her medication, however, until Abuzzahab enrolled her in a trial of an experimental antipsychotic drug. In the trial, she was taken off her regular medication, and she became suicidal. When Abuzzahab gave her a day pass to leave the hospital unsupervised, she threw herself into the Mississippi River and drowned. In another case cited by the board, Abuzzahab had prescribed a "large supply of potentially lethal medications" to a woman with a history of substance abuse, "shortly after a serious suicide attempt." She committed suicide by taking an overdose.[13]

The public portion of Abuzzahab's disciplinary file is freely available from the Minnesota licensing board and has been posted on the Web site of CIRCARE, a watchdog group that documents research abuse. When I ran a Google search for *Faruk Abuzzahab,* the first hit I got was a 1998 article in the *Globe* on his drug-trial disasters. Yet none of this seems to have derailed Abuzzahab's research career. Even after his suspension, he continued to supervise drug trials and to receive payments from at least a dozen drug companies.[14] In 2003, the American Psychiatric Association awarded him a Distinguished Life Fellowship.

The U.S. regulatory system is built on the tacit assumption that the main threat to research subjects comes from overly ambitious academic researchers who might be tempted to gamble with subjects' health in the pursuit of medical knowledge or academic fame. The system was intended to check this sort of intellectual ambition, primarily by ensuring that studies are reviewed in advance by boards made up of the researchers' academic peers. But like most physicians supervising clinical trials today, Abuzzahab does not work in an academic setting. The studies conducted at for-profit sites such as Prism are not the natural domain of academically ambitious researchers. The results are rarely published, and even if they were, they would bring little intellectual credit to the physicians carrying them out because they are designed by the industry sponsor. A researcher like Abuzzahab would not become famous by supervising subjects in studies like these. But he might become rich.

Abuzzahab represents a new, entrepreneurial breed of physician-researcher; in fact, many of his colleagues have moved even farther from the academic realm. In 1994, according to the Tufts Center for Drug Development, 70 percent of clinical researchers were affiliated with academic medical centers; by 2006 that figure had dropped to 36 percent.[15] The work can be lucrative, and some sponsors offer researchers additional financial incentives to recruit subjects. One doctor told the Department of Health and Human Services that he was offered twelve thousand dollars for each subject that he could enroll in a trial, plus a thirty-thousand-dollar bonus and an additional six thousand dollars per subject after the first six.

Some of the people directing clinical trials have little training in how to conduct research. And, as the Abuzzahab case suggests, not all drug companies are especially selective about the researchers they hire. In 2001, the FDA asked the pharmaceutical company Sanofi-Aventis to perform new studies of the antibiotic Ketek, which was suspected of causing liver failure. Reports later revealed that the top-recruiting investigator hired by PPD, the firm contracted by Sanofi-Aventis to conduct the studies, was a graduate of an offshore medical school who tested the antibiotic on clients in an obesity clinic she ran in Alabama. She was sentenced to five years in federal prison for fraud. Another top-recruiting investigator was arrested when the police found him carrying a loaded semiautomatic handgun and hiding cocaine in his underwear.[16]

Economics are also pushing trials to unexpected places. Drug firms have a much easier time finding willing subjects in the developing world, where medical facilities are crumbling and health-care budgets are minuscule. Subjects there may enroll in drug studies simply because that may be their only opportunity for any medical treatment whatsoever. By 2004, according to the Food and Drug Administration, drug companies were launching more than sixteen hundred new trials a year overseas.[17] In 2005, 40 percent of all trials were carried out in emerging markets. Eastern and Central Europe were early popular locations for trials. From 1995 to 2006, the largest annual increases in the number of clinical investigators carrying out trials were in Russia, India, Argentina, Poland, Brazil, and China.[18]

Some of these trials have been disastrous. In 1996, Trovan (trovafloxacin) was an investigational antibiotic that had shown promise against a broad range of infections and that could be administered in oral form instead of by injection. When news broke of a deadly meningitis epidemic in Nigeria, Pfizer flew a team of researchers to the industrial city of Kano to conduct a quick trial of Trovan on afflicted children. Pfizer set up shop next to the relief group Doctors Without Borders, which was desperately attempting to treat the meningitis victims, and quickly tested Trovan on two hundred children; half of them received Trovan and half received ceftriaxone, a proven treatment for meningitis when given in the proper dosage. Eleven children died, five of whom had taken Trovan and six of whom had taken ceftriaxone. According to the Nigerian families, many other children became blind, deaf, brain-damaged, or paralyzed.[19] When the study was finished, the Pfizer team abruptly returned home.

A Nigerian government report investigating the Kano study mysteriously disappeared; in 2006 it suddenly surfaced and was leaked to the press. According to the report, Pfizer never informed the parents, much less the children, that the treatment was part of an experiment. A letter of approval from a Nigerian ethics committee, which Pfizer used to justify its actions, apparently had been concocted and backdated by the company's primary researcher in Kano. Even more alarming were allegations brought against Pfizer by a number of Nigerian families. According to these allegations, not only did the Pfizer researchers fail to rescue desperately ill children whose condition was clearly deteriorating, they also gave the children in the control arm of the trial an inadequate dose of ceftriaxone, presumably in order to make Trovan look better by comparison. If this is true, the success of Trovan in the trial was won at the expense of the lives of the undertreated children. In 2009, Pfizer settled a lawsuit with the Nigerian government for seventy-five million dollars. [20]

The ease with which drug companies can test drugs overseas has simply ratcheted up the financial pressures on local investigators who want to keep trials at home. Now even university departments must compete with private companies. But as Marcia Angell, the former editor of the *New England Journal of Medicine,* has pointed out, competing with the private sector means doing trials under conditions set by private industry.[21] Those conditions are leading university researchers into ethically treacherous territory.

· · ·

Not too long ago, on a rainy May afternoon, I drove out to Cottage Grove, Minnesota, a suburb of St. Paul, to visit a woman named Mary Weiss. Mary and I had met a year or so earlier, after I learned that her son, Dan, had committed suicide in a psychiatric clinical trial at the University of Minnesota. Two journalists at the *St. Paul Pioneer Press,* Paul Tosto and Jeremy Olson, had investigated Dan's death, and what they described was deeply unsettling. In the months after the *Pioneer Press* story I talked informally to several university colleagues and administrators. Most of them dismissed the story as slanted and incomplete. Yet the more I looked into the circumstances surrounding Dan's death, the more convinced I became that something had gone badly wrong.

Mary Weiss is a slight, gray-haired woman, given to dressing in jeans and sweaters. She has a way of smiling ruefully at nearly any question, no matter how painful. When Dan was a child, Mary told me, the two of them lived in south St. Paul, an only child and a single mother. Dan was an easy, intelligent child, and as Mary showed me some old photographs, I could see how he had grown into his good looks. An excellent student, Dan had graduated from the University of Michigan in 2000 and moved to Los Angeles, hoping to become a screenwriter. To support himself in Los Angeles, he got a job as a celebrity-tour-bus driver.

In the summer of 2003, Mary went out to Los Angeles for a visit. She soon became alarmed by Dan's strange behavior. "When he picked me up, he said, 'You haven't told me when the event is going to be,'" Mary says. But Mary had no idea what event Dan was talking about. The next day Dan took her to his condo. "He was showing me a magazine, and showing me these numbers, which to him had a lot of significance, and he expected they did for me too, and they didn't." Later Dan pointed out a spot on the carpet in his apartment, which he claimed had been burned there by aliens. When I asked Mary how she reacted to all of this she replied, "I panicked."

Mary eventually convinced Dan to come back with her to St. Paul. She was certain that Dan was not just mentally ill but also potentially dangerous. His delusions revolved around a satanic cult orchestrating an "event" in Duluth at which Dan would be called upon to murder people, including Mary. Eventually Mary got so alarmed she called the St. Paul police. Dan was taken to Regions Hospital in St. Paul on November 12, where he was given Risperdal (risperidone), an antipsychotic drug often prescribed for patients with schizophrenia or bipolar disorder. The hospital had no psychiatric beds available, so Dan was transferred to Fairview Hospital, a teaching hospital for the University of Minnesota, where he was seen by Dr. Stephen Olson, a faculty member in the Department of Psychiatry. Olson believed that Dan was psychotic and dangerous; on November 14 he recommended that Dan be involuntarily committed to a state mental institution. Five days later an independent clinical psychologist also recommended involuntary commitment, explaining that Dan had threatened to slit his mother's throat.

Involuntary commitment is a legal procedure reserved for patients who are both mentally ill and dangerous to themselves or others. But in Minnesota, patients who have been involuntarily committed are given another option: a stay of commitment. This means that patients can avoid commitment as long as they agree to comply with the treatment recommendations of their psychiatrists. On November 20 Olson recommended a stay of commitment, telling the court that Dan had begun to admit that he needed help. The court agreed and ordered Dan to follow Olson's recommendations. The next day, Olson invited Dan to take part in an industry-funded drug study that he was conducting. Dan signed a consent form and was enrolled in the study immediately.

When Mary found out, she was stunned and upset. She had brought

Dan to Fairview for treatment, not a drug study, and she did not believe that Dan was mentally capable of understanding what he was agreeing to do. In fact, both Olson and the second clinician had judged him mentally incapable of consenting to antipsychotic medication. (In Minnesota, any patient treated with antipsychotic drugs must sign a written consent form. Dan was not asked to sign.) It was unclear how Dan could be judged incapable of consenting to treatment with antipsychotic drugs but capable of consenting to research with the same drugs—especially when the alternative to consenting appeared to be involuntary commitment.

The study, which was designed to last a full year, was funded by AstraZeneca and given the acronym *CAFE,* for "Comparison of Atypicals in First Episode." It was aimed at patients experiencing their first psychotic break. The CAFE study compared three different atypical antipsychotic drugs, each of which was already on the market: Seroquel (quetiapine), Zyprexa (olanzapine), and Risperdal (risperidone). The study was blinded, which meant that neither Dan nor Olson would know which drug he was taking; it was also randomized, which meant that Dan would be randomly assigned by computer to a study drug.

After Dan was enrolled in the study, he stayed at Fairview for about two more weeks. On December 8, he was transferred to Theo House, a halfway house in St. Paul. Olson thought Dan's symptoms were under control, but Mary was still very worried. She recalls a meeting with Olson at Fairview. "Olson came in and sat down and opened his file and said, 'Oh, Dan is doing so well.' And I said, 'No, Dr. Olson, Dan is not doing well.' I think he was taken aback."

At the halfway house Dan became more reclusive, often isolating himself in his room for days. He lost weight and stopped changing his clothes. His clinicians said they saw improvement, but Mary thought he was getting worse—angrier and more agitated. Dan kept a daily journal that shows his worsening mental state, according to Mike Howard, a family friend. "In his journal he kept, once he got to Theo House, his beliefs, and his illness did not get any better," Mike says. "It got worse. There is absolutely zero improvement." Over the following months Mary tried everything she could think of to get Dan out of the study. She called Olson and went to see him in the hospital but was unable to get a response. She wrote five letters to Olson and Dr. Charles Schulz, the chairman of the Department of Psychiatry and a co-investigator on the CAFE study, expressing her concern about Dan's condition, especially his inner rage. She received only one reply, from Schulz, who wrote that "it was not clear to me how you thought the treatment team should deal with this issue." Finally, in April 2004, Mary left a voice message with the study coordinator, asking, "Do we have to wait until he kills himself or someone else before anyone does anything?"

Three weeks later, Dan stabbed himself to death with a utility knife, slicing his throat and ripping open his abdomen. His body was discovered in the shower by a halfway house worker, along with a note on the nightstand that said *I went through this experience smiling*. When the blind on the study was broken, researchers found that Dan was being treated with Seroquel, the drug manufactured by AstraZeneca.

Suicide can be as hard to predict as it is to understand. If a patient with schizophrenia kills himself while taking an antipsychotic drug, was the suicide the result of the schizophrenia or of the drug? Schizophrenia heightens the risk of suicide and violence, and for this reason, most studies testing antipsychotic drugs specifically exclude patients at risk of killing themselves or other people.[22] Which raises this question: why was Dan, who had been recommended for involuntary commitment precisely because he had the psychotic delusion that he was being called on to commit murder, recruited into such a study?

Olson told the *Pioneer Press* that even if Dan had not been enrolled in the CAFE study, he would have been treated with one of the three drugs being tested. Yet if Dan had not been in CAFE study, he and his treatment team would have known what drug he was taking, and his medication could have been changed if he was not doing well. His psychiatrist could also have added other drugs, or tried options that were not permitted by the study guidelines. But the CAFE study, like many such studies, had strict requirements about how subjects could be managed. Changing Dan's medications would have meant dropping him from the study and forfeiting a portion of the money being paid to the Department of Psychiatry for his participation.

This money remains one of the most disturbing aspects of the CAFE study. For each subject who completed the study, AstraZeneca paid the Department of Psychiatry $15,648. A portion of Olson's salary came from that money, as did the funding for other study personnel. In total, AstraZeneca paid the department $327,000 for the CAFE study. In addition, Olson had worked as a "thought leader" for AstraZeneca, giving paid talks as a member of its speakers' bureau. He had similar arrangements with Eli Lilly and Janssen, the makers of Zyprexa and Risperdal, respectively, the other drugs being tested. According to a database kept by the Minnesota pharmacy board, Olson received a total of $220,000 from the pharmaceutical industry, $160,000 of it from AstraZeneca. According to the same database, Charles Schulz, his co-investigator and the department chair, received $562,000 from industry, with $112,000 coming from AstraZeneca.

At the time Dan was enrolled in the CAFE study, the Department of Psychiatry had been getting pressure to recruit subjects. The University of Minnesota was an "underperforming site," according to AstraZeneca, and it had been put on probation for failing to recruit enough subjects. "We have definitely been struggling to get patients," said an e-mail from the study coordinator. According to its contract, the university was obliged to return the $15,648 per subject it was paid if it did not enroll a subject within eight weeks of receiving its study drug.

After Dan committed suicide, the death was investigated by the FDA, which did not assign any blame to the university or the study sponsor. The office of the state mental health ombudsman also looked into the case, but nothing came of its report. Mary eventually sued the University of Minnesota and AstraZeneca; the court dismissed the case with a summary judgment. The court did assign Olson a penalty of $75,000, but according to Mary, this was not even enough to cover the fees of the expert witnesses her attorney had hired.

When the results of the CAFE study were eventually published, in 2007, they showed little difference in the drugs being tested.[23] About 70 percent of subjects stopped taking their drugs, no matter which drug they had been assigned. Two years later, AstraZeneca announced that it would pay $520 million to settle two federal investigations and two whistle-blower lawsuits over its allegedly illegal marketing of Seroquel, which has been linked to diabetes and weight gain.[24] During that investigation, Charles Schulz, the co-investigator on the study in which Dan died, was forced to respond to evidence that he had hyped the benefits of Seroquel in a press release about a study comparing it with an older, less expensive drug. Internal documents at AstraZeneca showed that Seroquel had proven no better than the older drug, yet Schulz had praised Seroquel enthusiastically.[25]

Mary Weiss is a quiet woman, but her experience with the University of Minnesota has left her angry and bitter. It is not hard to see why. In the years since she lost her son she has written letters and filed complaints to one oversight body after the other, and at every turn she has gotten little but form letters, rejections, and dismissals. Even the articles in the *Pioneer Press* did not help. The University of Minnesota has been especially cold-blooded in its response, even by the standards of corporate bureaucracies. When the lawsuit over Dan's death was dismissed, the university filed a legal action demanding that Mary pay $57,000 to cover its legal expenses.

•   •   •

In 1902, Harvey Wiley, the chief of the Bureau of Chemistry in the Department of Agriculture—an office that would later become the FDA—was given five thousand dollars to study the effects of food preservatives on human health. At the time, there were virtually no limits on what chemicals a manufacturer could add to food. Nor was there much information on how dangerous those chemicals might be. Wiley set up a "hygienic table" in the basement of his department and fitted it out as a dining hall, complete with white tablecloths and a chef. Then he recruited volunteers to test the safety of the chemical-laced food. The volunteers, who were mainly medical students and aspiring scientists in the Department of Agriculture, agreed to eat only at mealtimes, submit to frequent medical exams, and carry around a satchel full of equipment to collect all their urine and feces. They become known as the Poison Squad.[26]

The first preservative the Poison Squad tested was borax. The initial dose of borax was very low, but as it was increased the volunteers began to have stomach pain and bowel trouble. Eventually they got headaches and experienced so much pain that they could no longer work. Later, the Poison Squad tested four other preservatives, three of which produced similar symptoms. No volunteers died, but according to Wiley, some of them contracted permanent impairments of the digestive system. Their work gave Wiley the ammunition he needed to ban the preservatives. "What is this grand movement for purity of food and drugs?" asked Wiley. "Only the application of ethics to digestion and therapeutics. This is the new philosophy. Namely, the morals of metabolism."[27] The work of Wiley and the Poison Squad eventually led to the passage of the Pure Food and Drug Act of 1906.

Drug testing has always involved a kind of moral trade-off in which subjects are asked to take risks for the good of other people. More often than one might expect, the subjects are perfectly willing to do it. Many are willing to take risks even when the good for others is abstract and impersonal—the health of the populace, the safety of the food supply, the advancement of science, the good of the country. Of course, the fact that people are so willing to act altruistically makes them vulnerable to exploitation. Scientific careerists or profit-seeking corporations may describe their research in misleadingly humanitarian terms as a way of recruiting well-intentioned volunteers. They might also look for volunteers in places where conditions make altruistic acts look especially appealing.

During World War II, for example, the Civilian Public Service (CPS) was set up as an alternative to the military for conscientious objectors, many of whom belonged to pacifist denominations such as the Quakers, the Mennonites, and the Brethren. Many CPS jobs involved menial labor, but another option for objectors was to volunteer for medical research, which was conducted at camps all over the United States. Some volunteers gargled pneumonia-infected sputum. Others wore lice-infested underwear in order to contract typhus. Another group of participants allowed mosquito-filled boxes to be strapped to their bellies so that they would get malaria. And as Todd Tucker documents in his book *The Great Starvation Experiment,* one famous group of subjects at the University of Minnesota was intentionally starved.[28]

The Minnesota study was conducted toward the end of the World War II in order to understand how best to treat malnourished citizens in the newly liberated countries of Eastern Europe. The experiment's chief scientist, Ancel Keys, placed thirty-six young men on semi-starvation rations for six months. The subjects emerged looking like concentration-camp victims, but the most unexpected risks came from the psychological effects of starvation: the slow narrowing of desire, the obsession with food, the disturbing dreams of cannibalism. One subject wound up "accidentally" chopping off his fingers with an ax so that he would be dropped from the trial.

Today the CPS medical studies are not generally considered scandalous. In fact, Keys has been widely celebrated. This is not because anyone believes the CPS subjects were well treated. The government did not pay them for their work. (As Tucker points out, even German POWs received eighty cents a day.) If CPS volunteers were killed or disabled during their service, they got no compensation. Overall, thirty people died in CPS camps, and fifteen hundred were discharged without compensation for disabilities. Yet the CPS subjects understood the starvation study and were proud to take part. In fact, the rigors of the study were precisely what gave the experiment such an appeal. The stigma of being a conscientious objector was the accusation of cowardice, and according to some CPS subjects, the starvation study was a way to demonstrate bravery without picking up a gun.

Guinea-pigging for the CPS was exceptional, of course. It carried the air of a patriotic mission. In the age of corporate-funded mass drug production, most people feel little personal stake in the research enterprise and even less trust in the pharmaceutical industry that funds it. Not many people feel a moral duty to take part in these studies. "The reality is that we are not working for some noble cause," says James Rockwell. "This is about pharmaceutical companies developing as many drugs as fast as they can to make as much money as they can."

• • •

In early December of 2002, a man named Bob Helms took part in an industry-sponsored drug-delivery study. Helms and his fellow guinea pigs were required to take a new antianxiety drug and, later, to defecate into a small basket. The unfortunate clinic staff members then searched for the remains of the tablet to determine how much had been absorbed by the body.

The guinea pigs were each paid thirty-three hundred dollars and were required to live in the unit for five four-day periods. But before the end of the first period, Helms says, the guinea pigs decided that they were getting a raw deal. The process of fecal collection was smelly and unpleasant; the amount of time allowed outside the unit had been shortened from three days to thirty-six hours; and the subjects were required to abstain from alcohol, even though the study—because of unexpected delays—was taking place over the Christmas and New Year's holidays. The guinea pigs wanted a raise.

Since the staff was collecting their feces, Helms suggested that the guinea pigs all swallow notes that said *More money*. This idea was rejected. Instead, they presented a one-page memo to the staff detailing their concerns and requesting a pay increase of eleven hundred dollars. When the memo was ignored, they began hinting that they might decamp for a better-paying study at another site. Eventually, the clinic agreed to pay each subject an additional eight hundred dollars.

Helms is a pioneer in the world of guinea-pig activism. A fifty-one-year-old housepainter and former union organizer, he has a calm, measured demeanor that masks a deep dissident streak. Before he started guinea-pigging, in the 1990s, he worked as a caregiver for mentally retarded adults living in group homes. There Helms began to understand the difficulties in organizing health-care workers who were employed by a single company but who worked in far-flung locations—in this case, group homes that were spread over two hundred miles of suburbs. "The other organizers told me right off the bat that I could not organize workers who might meet each other once a year at best," Helms says. "How could we ask them to take risks together? They were strangers." Helms saw that guinea pigs faced a similar problem, and in 1996 he started a jobzine for research subjects, called *Guinea Pig Zero*.

The look of *Guinea Pig Zero* was rough and handmade, as if it had been stapled together with paper stolen from Kinko's, and many issues featured an actual guinea pig on the cover. The writing sounded like a cross between Emma Goldman and Robert Crumb. One early issue ran an article about donating eggs to a fertility clinic. It had the title "Cluck, Cluck, Gimme a Buck." A cartoon in an early issue shows a young man surrounded by IV bags and syringes exclaiming, "No more fast food work for me—I've got a career in science!" The contrast between the language of *Guinea Pig Zero* and that of a clinical-research protocol could not have been more dramatic. Research protocols call subjects "research participants." *Guinea Pig Zero* called them "medical meat-puppets" or "brain sluts." The protocols pretend that people enroll in studies to advance science. *Guinea Pig Zero* assumed that nobody in his right mind would enroll in a study for anything but the money. The protocols described the risk and discomforts of studies in oblique clinical language. *Guinea Pig Zero* was more direct. "The physicians you'll meet will throw in the old prostate exam, just for the hell of it," wrote Helms in one issue. "But what's a finger up the ass between friends?"

Each issue featured a section called "The Treadmill of History," in which Helms wrote about research abuses and disasters over the ages, but the most compelling parts of the 'zine were the firsthand accounts from Helms and his guinea-pig field reporters. With a mixture of advocacy and dark humor, *Guinea Pig Zero* published the sort of information that guinea pigs really wanted to know—how well a study paid, the competence of the venipuncturist, the quality of the food. It even published report cards, grading research units from A to F. "Overcrowding, no hot showers, sleeping in an easy chair, incredibly cheap shit for dinner, creepy guys from New York jails—all these are a poor man's worries," Helms says. "Where are these things in the regulators' paperwork?" In one issue a guinea pig identified as Donno wrote about a sleep-deprivation study at the University of Pennsylvania where his mental condition deteriorated so much that he began to hallucinate that he was Tony Randall guest-hosting *The Tonight Show*. Theresa Dulce, a guinea pig reporting from PPD Pharmaco in Austin, Texas, was identified as "the editrix of Danzine, the smart & sexy journal by and for ladies in the sex business." Her article was titled "Spanish Fly Guinea Pig" and appeared with a photograph of a near-naked woman wearing a G-string and a pig nose. At PPD Pharmaco, Dulce wrote, "Every meal created a new challenge in how to get rid of unwanted gruel. One guy put a pork chop in his sock, walking out of the cafeteria to flush it down in little pieces."[29] In a report on SmithKline Beecham, Helms wrote about a psychiatric drug study where a guinea pig "emerged from the unit with $7,000 in his pocket and his mind on planet Zork."

Guinea Pig Zero was not aimed at sick people who sign up for studies in order to get new treatment. It was aimed at poor people who sign up for studies in order to get money. And here is where its perspective diverged most radically from the traditional ethical perspective. *Guinea Pig Zero* assumed that subjects should get more money, while many ethicists and regulators argued that they should get none at all.

The standard worry expressed by ethicists is that money tempts subjects to take part in dangerous, painful, or degrading studies against their better judgment. FDA guidelines instruct review boards to make sure that payment is not "coercive" and does not exert an "undue influence" on subjects. It's a reasonable worry. "If there were a study where they cut off your leg and sewed it back on and you got twenty thousand dollars, people would be fighting to get into that study," a Philadelphia activist and clinical-trial veteran who writes under the name Dave Onion says.

Of course, ethicists generally prefer that subjects take part in studies for altruistic reasons. Yet if sponsors relied solely on altruism, studies on healthy subjects would probably come to a halt. The result is an uneasy compromise: guinea pigs are paid to test drugs, but everyone pretends that guinea-pigging is not really a job. IRBs allow sponsors to pay guinea pigs but, consistent with FDA guidelines, insist on their keeping the amount low. Sponsors refer to the money as "compensation" rather than "wages," but guinea pigs must pay taxes, and they are given no retirement benefits, disability insurance, workers' compensation, or overtime pay. And, because so many guinea pigs are uninsured, they are testing the safety of drugs that they will probably not be able to afford once the drugs have been approved. "I'm not going to get the benefit of the health care that is developed by this research," Helms says, "because I am not in the economic class to get health insurance."

Guinea pigs can't even count on having their medical care paid for if they are injured in a study. According to a recent survey in the *New England Journal of Medicine,* only 16 percent of academic medical centers in the United States provided free care to subjects injured in trials. None of them compensated injured subjects for pain or lost wages.[30] No systematic data are available for private testing sites, but the provisions typically found in consent forms are not encouraging. A consent form for a recent study of Genentech's immunosuppressant drug Raptiva told participants that they would be treated for any injuries the drug caused but stipulated that "the cost of such treatment will not be reimbursed."

Some sponsors withhold most of the payment until the studies are over. Guinea pigs who drop out after deciding that a surgical procedure is too disagreeable or that a drug seems unpleasant or dangerous must forfeit the bulk of their paychecks. Two years ago, when SFBC conducted a two-month study of the pain medication Palladone, it offered subjects twenty-four hundred dollars. But most of that was paid only after the last of the study's four confinement periods. A guinea pig could spend nearly two months in the study, including twelve days and nights in the SFBC unit, and get only six hundred dollars. SFBC even reserved the right to withhold payments from subjects whom it dropped from the study because of a drug's side effects.

Guinea-pig activists recognize that they are indispensable to the pharmaceutical industry; a guinea-pig walkout in the middle of a trial could wreak financial havoc on the sponsor. Yet the conditions of guinea-pigging make any exercise of power difficult. Not only are those in a particular trial likely to be strangers to one another, but if they complain to the sponsor about conditions, they risk being excluded from future studies. And according to *Bloomberg Markets,* when illegal-immigrant guinea pigs at SFBC talked to the press, managers threatened to have them deported.[31]

Lawsuits on behalf of injured subjects are growing, though, and they have begun to target not just research sponsors but also institutional review boards and bioethicists. Alan Milstein, an attorney in Philadelphia, has pioneered this area of law, most notably with successful litigation against the University of Pennsylvania on behalf of the family of Jesse Gelsinger, who died in a gene-therapy trial in 1999. Milstein has represented volunteers injured at commercial sites, but most guinea pigs are in no position to hire a lawyer. "This is not something you or I do," Milstein says. "This is something the poor do so that the rich can get better drugs."

• • •

During our early years of medical school, my classmates and I were given a course in physical diagnosis. Usually, we practiced on one another. Each of us would percuss a classmate's chest or listen to his heart with a stethoscope. But some procedures were considered too personal to practice on a classmate. For some of these, we were assigned a "model patient"—someone from the community who was "compensated" in exchange for undergoing an examination.

This was how I performed my first rectal exam. A large group of us were led into a room where our model patient was bent over an examining table with his pants around his ankles. One by one, we approached him nervously from behind, inserted a gloved, lubricated finger into his rectum, and felt around for the prostate. "Thank you," we all said politely to the model patient as we removed our index fingers from his anus. The model patient stared straight ahead, saying nothing.

What made the experience oddly disturbing was not just the forced, pseudo normality of the instruction or the fact that the exam could have been done more privately, but the instrumentality of the encounter: a pretend patient bending over naked for anonymous strangers in exchange for money. The fact that the model patient had been paid did not make his work seem any less degrading. (Tipping him would have made it even worse.)

Perhaps there is something inherently disconcerting about the idea of turning drug testing into a job. Guinea pigs do not do things in exchange for money so much as they allow things to be done to them. There are not many other jobs where that is the case. Meanwhile, our patchwork regulatory system insures that no single institution is keeping track of how many deaths and injuries befall healthy subjects in clinical trials. Nobody appears to be tracking how many clinical investigators are incompetent, or have lost their licenses, or have questionable disciplinary records. Nobody is monitoring the effect that so many trials have on the health of professional guinea pigs. In fact, nobody is even entirely certain whether the trials generate reliable data. A professional guinea pig who does a dozen drug-safety trials a year is not exactly representative of the population that will be taking the drugs once they have been approved.

The safety of new drugs has always depended on the willingness of someone to test them, and it seems inevitable that the job will fall to people who have no better options. Guinea-pigging requires no training or skill, and in a thoroughly commercial environment, where there can be no pretense of humanitarian motivation, it is hard to think of it as meaningful work. As Dave Onion puts it, "You don't go home and say to yourself, 'Now, that was a good day.'"

CHAPTER TWO

The Ghosts

TEN YEARS AGO, when David Bronstein finished his PhD in developmental biology, he was at a loss for what to do with the degree. Ordinarily the next step would have been a postdoctoral fellowship. But Bronstein had been working in the laboratory long enough to suspect that he was not that good at bench science, and in any case, he did not especially enjoy it. One day his father showed him a newspaper advertisement. A medical communications agency was looking for a trained medical writer. Bronstein was hired on the spot, even though he had no idea what a medical communications agency actually did.

Bronstein (a pseudonym) is a lanky Englishman in his midforties. His manner is wry and self-deprecating, and something about him seems jaded and world-weary, like a character from a Graham Greene novel. His first assignment at the agency was to produce scientific abstracts for studies of a newly approved antibiotic. Unfortunately, the antibiotic had a major flaw: it did not work against pneumococcus. Pneumococcus is one of the most common bugs that a doctor sees; it is responsible for a fair bit of pneumonia and meningitis. But this flaw was not something that the drug's manufacturer—which was funding the articles and abstracts—was keen to point out. So Bronstein and the other writers were told that they should simply avoid the topic. Bronstein compares the instruction to a famous episode of the British sitcom *Fawlty Towers* in which Basil Fawlty has guests coming from Germany and keeps telling the staff: "Don't mention the war!" At the agency, says Bronstein, the running joke was "Don't mention the pneumococcus!"

Drug marketing is a complicated affair. It is subject to a complex regulatory apparatus; it concerns technically arcane, potentially dangerous products; and for most of its history, it has been aimed not at the patients who will buy and use the medications but at the doctors who prescribe them. These constant pressures and constraints have forced the marketing down unusual paths. Like a hardy plant that has been grown in a dark, confined space, drug marketing has developed into a highly resilient but peculiarly shaped organism whose branches extend in unexpected directions, searching for light. It goes without saying that most drug marketing is not supposed to look like marketing. Doctors insist (and patients want to believe) that they prescribe drugs based on empirical evidence, not on advertisements. So from the very start, drugmakers have tried to design marketing tools that resemble, as closely as possible, the vehicles that transmit empirical evidence: medical journals, scientific articles, abstracts, symposia, conferences, slide shows, and grand-rounds presentations. Until recently, even drug reps managed a pretty decent impression of scientific expertise.

It was this impression of scientific expertise that almost fooled Bronstein. On the surface, it appeared as if his new job would not be all that different from what he was used to doing as an academic biologist. Biologists write up abstracts of their work; they send off articles to scientific journals; they make PowerPoint presentations to show their peers at distant conferences. Bronstein was doing all these things at the agency, but he did it at the bidding of a drugmaker with a marketing agenda. Critics would call Bronstein a ghostwriter, and it is true that he wrote articles that were later published under the names of prominent academic physicians, usually with no mention of his involvement. But the term *ghostwriter* suggests a much higher degree of literary creativity than what the job actually entailed. Bronstein's job did not resemble what Ted Sorensen did for John Kennedy as much as it resembled what a writer of computer instruction manuals does for Microsoft. He produced highly technical, stylized publications and slide kits that looked, at least at first, like the standard materials of scientific communication. Bronstein left the agency after a year, but he still works as a freelance medical writer and consultant. When I asked him how long it took him to decide that there was something ethically dubious going on at the agency, he replied, "The first day I was there."

• • •

It is hard to pinpoint exactly when the business of medical communications began. This is partly because the business is made up of projects that drug companies used to do themselves but now outsource to others, and partly because the concept of medical communications is so amorphous. Some agencies call themselves medical education companies, while others, especially in the United Kingdom, say they are in the business of health-care public relations. Some agencies are owned by multinational advertising companies; others are small, independent shops with only a handful of employees. Very few agencies have been around for longer than twenty-five years. In the United States, the niche for medical communications widened dramatically in the 1990s, when policy changes started to make it difficult for pharmaceutical companies to produce their own educational materials. By 2008, 144 medical education and communications agencies were operating in the United States, many of them concentrated in the northeastern urban corridor around Philadelphia, New York, and New Jersey, where a number of drug companies are headquartered.[1] Despite their growing importance, the agencies are still so unfamiliar to most people in academic medicine that nobody seems quite sure what they are called. Some people use the acronym *MECC*, for "medical education and communications companies," or they use *MESS*, for "medical education service suppliers." Perhaps the most common terms are abbreviations such as *med comms* and *med ed companies*.

In the business of medical communications, the term *medical education* covers a lot of ground. Most agencies work at least in part for the pharmaceutical and medical-device industries, for which they produce a whole range of educational and communications materials, from magazine articles and slide kits to podcasts and Webinars. Many agencies organize grand-rounds lectures at hospitals, recruiting speakers and preparing their slides. Some agencies help pharmaceutical companies train "opinion leaders" and manage their speakers' bureaus. Most of them organize a number of live events, such as satellite symposia at conferences and advisory board meetings.

A good proportion of this material is officially accredited as Continuing Medical Education (CME) for physicians.[2] Accredited CME has an enviable market niche; most physicians are required to take part in a certain number of CME events in order to maintain their licenses to practice. In the old days, CME was produced by universities and professional societies, and it was largely paid for by registration fees and the groups that were sponsoring it. Over time, however, the proportion of CME that is funded by the pharmaceutical and device industries has crept steadily upward. The sharpest uptick has occurred over the past ten years or so. Between 1998 and 2006, commercial support for CME increased by a fourfold margin to a total of $1.2 billion. By 2006, over 60 percent of CME was funded by commercial sources. During this same period, profit margins for accredited CME providers increased nearly sixfold, from 5.5 percent to 31 percent, with total income reaching $2.38 billion.[3]

The official body charged with ensuring that CME is unbiased is the Accreditation Council for Continuing Medical Education (ACCME). ACCME certifies certain bodies as accredited CME providers; in turn, those accredited CME providers are given the authority to certify CME events as credits toward the fulfillment of professional educational requirements. ACCME-accredited providers include the CME offices of universities and professional societies, but they also include medical communications agencies and, in one case, a pharmaceutical company. Accredited CME providers have a financial interest in maintaining the goodwill of the providers whose events they are accrediting. For instance, when a university CME office accredits a CME event, it will usually take a small cut of the funding—typically 5 to 7 percent—in accreditation fees. Today, even university CME offices get the majority of their income from the pharmaceutical and medical-device industries, although their profit margins are lower than medical communications agencies'.[4]

One growing arm of this increasingly lucrative business is the management and production of scientific articles. The term of art for this activity is *publication planning.* The business of publication planning established itself during the 1990s, as industry profits were escalating and clinical research was moving out of academic health centers and into contract research organizations. Publication planning is seen as essential to the marketing plan for any new drug and it begins years in advance of a launch. Publication planners will help a pharmaceutical company design scientific articles that reinforce a larger marketing plan—or, as one agency puts it, help them "connect data to key messages to support product positioning." (That agency's slightly creepy slogan: "Weaving the web of evidence.")[5] Publication planners will ask how a new drug differs from other drugs on the market, which practitioners need to be reached, and what sort of scientific journals should be targeted. They will debate the finer points of general journals versus specialty journals, letters versus articles, peer-reviewed journals versus throwaways, and the merits of industry-sponsored journal supplements. The details of publication planning can sound arcane to outsiders, yet the business has become large enough to support two international professional societies: an industry-run organization called the International Publication Planning

Association, and a nonprofit group, the International Society for Medical Publication Professionals.

The scientific publications themselves are produced by professional medical writers, many of whom have backgrounds in science. Some medical communications agencies have their own teams of writers, as do some pharmaceutical companies, but many agencies simply contract the work out to freelancers. According to a 2005 article in the *Wall Street Journal*, a medical writer can usually expect to be paid $90 to $120 per hour. [6] A survey by the American Medical Writers Association in 2006 found that the average freelance medical writer in the United States made close to $120,000 per annum, and writers with graduate education beyond a master's degree made close to $150,000.[7]

The mechanics of ghostwriting are fairly simple.[8] According to Bronstein, the agency starts by liaising with the marketers and other interested parties in the drug company. First they will agree on a title for the article. Next they will decide on a potential "author," usually an academic physician with a reputation as a thought leader or opinion leader. The purpose of recruiting an academic physician to sign on as author is to give the article more legitimacy; physicians are less likely to trust an article if its author works for a pharmaceutical company. (The same goes for conference presentations, satellite symposia, and academic lectures.) The physician is contacted by the agency and asked if he or she would be willing to "author" the article, often in exchange for a fee. Fees generally range from $1,000 to $2,500 per article. If the author agrees to sign on, a brief, or a set of instructions, will be prepared for the ghostwriter. The ghostwriter will write either the full article or an extended outline; this will be reviewed by the agency and the drug company and then sent on to the author. The author may ask for changes, or may simply approve the article as written. Once everyone agrees on a suitable version of the article and it has received legal approval, the author will submit the article to a journal, where, if all goes well, it will be published. Generally the work of the medical writer and the agency goes unmentioned, unless they are thanked in the acknowledgments section for writing assistance. Bronstein rarely even sees the published articles he has written. In fact, he says, the articles can be pretty hard to track down.

No one knows for certain how much of the medical literature is ghostwritten. For many years, ghostwriting was assumed to be rare. Until fairly recently, the best-known article on ghostwriting was a survey published in the *Journal of the American Medical Association* in 1998, which found evidence of ghost authorship in 11 percent of articles published in six major American medical journals.[9] The results of that survey were hard to interpret, however, because the authors did not try to find out how many articles had originated with external organizations, such as medical education agencies or pharmaceutical companies.[10]

A hint of the actual figure emerged in a 2003 study in the *British Journal of Psychiatry* suggesting that the *JAMA* study may have dramatically underestimated the extent of industry involvement.[11] A lawsuit brought against Pfizer in 1999 had turned up documents produced by a medical communications company called Current Medical Directions, which had been working on a publications strategy for Pfizer's antidepressant Zoloft (sertraline). The documents listed all the Zoloft studies that Current Medical Directions had been preparing for publication in 1999, the journals where the papers had been submitted, the conferences where the papers had been presented, the authors of the articles, and so on. A clue that the articles were being ghosted came from the fact that for a number of already written articles the authors were listed as *TBD*, or "to be determined."

The authors of the *British Journal of Psychiatry* article, David Healy and Dinah Cattell, decided to track down the papers on Zoloft that Current Medical Directions had been working on and see what had happened to them. They picked three years (1998, 1999, and 2000) and searched the medical literature for all articles published on Zoloft during that time. What they found shocked many people. First, the agency-prepared articles outnumbered the articles written in the traditional way. Forty-one traditionally authored articles on Zoloft had been published, while fifty-five articles had come from Current Medical Directions. Second, the articles that came from Current Medical Directions had been published in far more prestigious journals than the traditionally authored articles. These articles ranged from *JAMA* through the *Archives of General Psychiatry* and the *American Journal of Psychiatry*. In fact, the citation rate for the Current Medical Directions' articles was over five times higher than the citation rate for the traditionally authored articles. Finally, the Current Medical Directions articles painted a much happier profile of Zoloft than did the traditionally authored articles. For example, the articles prepared by Current Medical Directions on pediatric psychopharmacology failed to mention five of the six children on Zoloft who took action toward committing suicide.

It is unclear how much can be concluded from the literature on a single drug. Yet litigation suggests that the strategy Pfizer and Current Medical Directions used to market Zoloft is not unusual. In fact, it is probably close to the norm. For instance, a marketing document uncovered during a Senate investigation revealed that in 2004, Forest Laboratories had budgeted $100,000 for ghostwritten articles on Lexapro.[12] (Lexapro is a me-too version of Forest's antidepressant Celexa; Forest introduced it when Celexa was going off-patent as a way of keeping profits flowing.) Similarly, in 2009, court documents revealed that Wyeth (now part of Pfizer) had paid ghostwriters to produce twenty-six articles backing the use of its hormone replacement drugs Prempro and Premarin, even after evidence showed that the drugs caused an increased risk of breast cancer, heart disease, and stroke.[13] Litigation against Eli Lilly in 2008 showed that Lilly had hired ghostwriters to promote its antipsychotic Zyprexa, a drug that has become controversial because of its links to obesity and diabetes.[14]

Perhaps the most brazen ghostwriting campaign was that of GlaxoSmithKline, which came under fire for its promotion of the antidepressant Paxil as safe and non-habit-forming when evidence had linked the drug to an increased risk of suicidal ideation in children.[15] In 2004 GSK settled a legal action by the New York attorney general for $2.5 million. Later, it emerged that GlaxoSmithKline had promoted Paxil through a novel ghostwriting program aimed at recruiting physicians to "author" case studies. It was called Case Study Publications for Peer Review, which the company usefully shortened to the acronym CASPPER.[16]

•　　•　　•

To many critics, the main problem with medical ghostwriting is that academic physicians get credit for articles that they didn't actually write. The status of any academic depends heavily on his or her scholarship, and in academic medicine, the most important measure of scholarship is the sheer quantity of articles produced. The more papers a physician authors, the higher he or she elevates in the academic hierarchy. And if an academic physician is not actually doing the work behind the papers but is simply signing articles written by agency-employed medical writers, that physician's taking credit for the paper seems scandalous, like a student who buys a paper on the Internet. "I don't feel really good about ghostwriting an article that is going to appear under the name of a doctor at Brown University who is going to get twenty-five hundred dollars to do nothing more than review it," says Susan Gilbert, a writer who worked briefly for a medical communications agency before going into bioethics. "The whole structure of the business was wrong to me."

The practice of ghostwriting is rediscovered every few years by investigative reporters, often when a drug scandal breaks. These investigative reports are generally written with the assumption that a reader will understand right away exactly what is wrong with medical ghostwriting. (In fact, the reports often leave readers with the impression that the practitioners will soon be led away in handcuffs and orange jumpsuits.) Yet this assumption is at striking odds with the attitudes of many physicians and medical education executives, who often seem quite bemused by all the fuss. They point out that most of the legitimate articles in medical journals have a number of authors, many of whom have done very little if any of the actual writing. Many academic physicians do not see a bright line between authoring articles with an education agency and authoring them with academic collaborators. Harry Sweeney, the head of a medical communications agency, puts it this way: "As research articles became more formulaic and less prosy, busy department heads used students and postdocs to draft their reports or formed medical writing groups to grind out the grants and publish-or-perish materials. So long as the putative 'author' reviews and edits a draft document, I find it difficult to see the problem."[17]

Sweeney has a point. It is a practice universally acknowledged, not always with pride, that the authors of legitimate, universally respected articles in academic medicine are not always the same people as those articles' writers. Sometimes this is completely understandable. Many research papers are genuinely collaborative projects, often with different tasks outsourced to various specialists—one to the epidemiologist, another to the clinician, yet another to the biostatistician, each of whom will be given an authorship credit on the resulting publication. Here, the authorship credit does not stand for writing but for intellectual contribution. According to one survey, only about 41 percent of authors of medical publications actually took part in writing the first draft of the article.[18]

But there is a lot of fuzziness in the notion of "intellectual contribution." In some academic units, for example, junior scholars are expected to list their department chairs or lab chiefs as coauthors on all their publications, whether or not these people have actually contributed anything to the paper. In fact, I have heard some senior academics argue that they should be listed as coauthors on anything written by anyone being paid out of their grants. The polite term for this is *honorary authorship* or *gift authorship*, a practice that is officially frowned upon by journal editors but that remains relatively common. A more benign version of honorary authorship is when a senior academic lists a junior partner (such as a graduate student or research assistant) as a coauthor on a publication out of generosity, even though that person has contributed very little. As a result, it can be difficult to look at the list of authors on a research paper and decode exactly who did what. An author may be the head of the department where the article was produced, or the person who wrote the grant that funded it, or simply a powerful senior physician to whom a junior academic has offered authorship in order to curry favor.

Some medical writers distinguish between ghost authoring and ghostwriting. "Ghost authoring is 'We write it, you sign it,' " says Michael Altus, a freelance medical writer. "Everyone condemns that." Ghostwriting, he says, is closer to a kind of joint authorship, where a writer collaborates with an author but without receiving any formal acknowledgment.[19] This practice is more controversial. Critics of ghostwriting say the lack of acknowledgment is an effort to hide the involvement of industry and make it appear as if the article has originated from a university. Defenders say that often the writer simply has not done enough intellectual work to be formally acknowledged. They see the work of a medical writer as similar to that of a secretary or, at best, an editor.

When it comes to authorship, different work cultures have different customs and practices. Nobody expects American politicians to write their own speeches anymore, and nobody expects celebrities to write their own memoirs. We listen to political speeches and read celebrity autobiographies with the same kind of ironic suspension of disbelief that we employ when we watch professional wrestling. In fact, quite a lot of the writing we read every day is not credited to anyone at all, even though someone somewhere must have written it: advertising copy, technical writing, the promotional descriptions on Web sites and book jackets. In the culture of academic medicine, accepting credit for a ghosted journal article is not seen as a serious ethical failing, simply because the skill of writing is not seen as a valuable intellectual talent.

In the humanities, writing a paper is regarded as genuine scholarly work. Writing an essay in philosophy or literary criticism is itself an act of creation, like writing a novel or a play. If we were to discover that Wittgenstein's *Tractatus*, for example, had been written by someone else, it would undermine everything we thought we knew about Wittgenstein the philosopher. But in science—and to some extent, in academic medicine—the serious intellectual work involved in producing an academic paper is not the act of writing. The serious work happens well in advance, when the study is being conceived, designed, and carried out. Writing up the results for a journal is important, but it is closer to a technical communication than a product of scholarship. Communicating the results is a little like court stenography—a skill that is not without standards of excellence but where excellence does not require intellectual creativity.

According to Bronstein, many critics of ghostwriting are aiming at the wrong target. "Ghosting seemed more of a personal humiliation, rather than a major moral crime," Bronstein says. Although it may be unfair for academic physicians to be promoted or tenured on the basis of articles they did not write, Bronstein considers this a minor sin compared to the commercial bias of the articles he was often asked to produce. As he says, "The moral crime I was being asked to commit was to do with truthfulness."

• • •

What we know (or think we know) about the world depends crucially on what others tell us about it. For science and medicine to work, scientists and physicians must be able to trust that what others tell them is true. Part of the reason science was able to take root as a way of understanding the world in the seventeenth century was the concept of the gentleman, who was bound by honor to be truthful. "Gentlemanly" culture involved social norms and conventions designed to promote truth-telling, such as the importance of face-to-face conversation. But the norms of gentlemanly culture clashed with those of the trading classes, where commercial imperatives strongly encouraged exaggeration and deception. As the historian Steven Shapin has observed, the gentle classes of the time "deplored the lying and deceit of merchants," even if they did not deplore the merchant activities themselves.[20]

This tension between science and commerce persists today. We still deplore the "lying and deceit" of merchants and rely on external bodies to regulate them, while we allow science to work on a kind of honor system. We simply trust scientists to tell the truth. The problem is that science itself is becoming more and more commercialized. Beginning in the 1980s, a series of legislative initiatives pushed science and commerce much closer together, especially the Bayh-Dole Act, which (among other things) gave universities the right to profit financially from their scientific research. The purpose of these initiatives was to bring scientific discoveries to market faster, but it also encouraged scientists to behave like entrepreneurs—or, as Shapin might have it, for gentlemen to behave like merchants.

Today, as Richard Horton, the editor of the *Lancet*, has pointed out, scientists are forced to compete with one another in the market.[21] They must treat their scientific data as a trade secret. As a result, scientists must waste money and effort duplicating the results of others. Often scientists cannot even investigate questions that are important to the public, or to science itself, but must instead investigate questions of concern to industry. Most important, competition gives industry-backed scientists incentives to stretch the truth.

"Manuscripts have to be framed in a certain way because of the spin that the company wants," says Linda Logdberg. Logdberg, like Bronstein, started her career as a scientist. By training, she is an anatomist. Logdberg stumbled into medical writing while she was working unhappily at a Columbia University affiliate hospital near New York. "It was a terrible job, weighing rats and cleaning rat cages," she says. "I worked with a crazed Orthodox Jew with a PhD in biochemistry who never bathed. He was very smart but he wouldn't give the police department his building security code to reset after he was robbed, because 'Why should I give my personal information to a goy?'" In 1991 Logdberg saw an ad in the *New York Times* for a medical writer. She left her research job and spent the next sixteen years as a writer, often working for medical communications agencies. For a time she worked with a company developing a birth control pill that prevented women from having menstrual periods. The company saw this as a big selling point—apparently, some women are happy not to have menstrual periods—but this pill had a problem. Some women taking it experienced severe menstrual bleeding two or three times a year. "My job was to turn this into a benefit," Logdberg says. "How do you turn severe unexpected bleeding into a benefit?"

It is easy to understand the pressure a company faces. What if you have invested millions of dollars in a drug, design a study to test it, and then the study turns out badly? You could simply go ahead and publish the study, of course, and present the data as honestly and objectively as possible. But that strategy might well be financially damaging to your company, especially if investors are skittish. So you might opt to postpone publication until later, or publish the study in a minor foreign journal where no one will notice it, or even simply not publish it at all. (Journals are notoriously less enthusiastic about publishing negative results anyway.) Alternatively, you could publish the study in a way that shows the poor results in a more positive light—by fiddling with the statistics, reclassifying side effects, or somehow spinning the results to suit your marketing goals. Logdberg refused to spin severe bleeding as a benefit, and the company never did submit their birth control pill for FDA approval.

David Bronstein believes that the decision to spin or bury data is usually less a matter of willful deceit than one of self-deception. "Everyone adopts a belief in the drug and becomes blind to the deficiencies," he says. Data are often ambiguous. Different studies often produce conflicting results, and even a single study is subject to different interpretations. When this happens, it becomes easier to convince yourself that something is wrong with a study, rather than the drug. "Is someone being unethical when they adopt an unreasonable belief?" Bronstein asks. Writers are in an especially tricky position, because their jobs depend on cultivating the goodwill of the companies that employ them. Bronstein says, "It is part of the game to present the drug the way they want it presented—otherwise you won't be hired."

Bronstein was once contracted to write publications for a drug that treated a heart disorder.[22] The drug worked well, except in one unexpected population: patients with advanced heart failure. In these patients, the drug could be dangerous. When the drug was tested against a placebo, patients with advanced heart failure who got the drug died more often than those with advanced heart failure who got the placebo. This finding made no sense, and the company researchers looked around for an explanation. Could it have something to do with the way doctors were managing heart failure patients? Might it be connected to another drug these particular patients were taking? Bronstein thought the data did not support this explanation, and eventually scientists within the company agreed. But excluding the use of the drug in patients with heart failure, especially those with mild heart failure, would place a major hurdle in the path to getting the drug approved by the FDA. Even if doctors were warned about prescribing the medication for patients who had advanced heart failure, the FDA was unlikely to approve a drug that might also be dangerous for patients with mild heart failure. The company did additional studies, but at this point Bronstein stopped working on the drug. When we last spoke, he was still unsure how the company would deal with the issue of mild heart failure in their published articles.

Original clinical studies are only one type of scientific publication that writers produce. They also write editorials, letters to the editor, and review articles, all of which may be published in peer-reviewed journals. These articles have an element of personal subjectivity that make them especially useful as promotional vehicles. Review articles, for example, summarize the current state of knowledge about an illness or a therapy based on the author's reading of the published literature. Because the entire point of a review article is to give nonexpert readers an expert's opinion, review articles can easily be framed in a way that is useful for a marketing department.

Pharmaceutical companies often publish review articles years before a drug is launched. The purpose of these articles is to prepare the ground for the drug's arrival—by pointing out the shortcomings of rival drugs, for example, or highlighting the seriousness of an under-recognized or undertreated illness for which their drug will later be presented as the remedy. The promotional aims of review articles can be difficult for an outsider to discern, which may be why opinion leaders often agree to "author" them. Adriane Fugh-Berman, a physician at Georgetown University who specializes in alternative and complementary medicine, was invited to author a review article produced by a medical education agency called Rx Communications.[23] The article, she was told, would be about the potential interactions between herbs and warfarin, an anticoagulant (or blood thinner). Suspicious of the agency's intentions, Fugh-Berman asked for more information. She was sent a completed manuscript with her name on it titled "Interactions Between Dietary Supplements and Warfarin: The Hazards of Self-Administration."

What puzzled Fugh-Berman was why a pharmaceutical company would fund a review article on the interaction between herbs and warfarin. What rationale could a drug company have for showing that such interactions might be dangerous? Fugh-Berman decided simply to ask Rx Communications. The agency told her that AstraZeneca, the sponsor of the article, was "keen to set the scene for new anticoagulants that are not subject to the numerous limitations of warfarin." AstraZeneca was developing its own anticoagulant, called Exanta, and planned to promote it by highlighting warfarin's drawbacks. "The thing I didn't know was that companies funded articles to kill a small part of the market," says Fugh-Berman. "I also didn't understand how far in advance of a drug launch they started seeding the literature."

Medical communications agencies also produce a tremendous amount of promotional work that is not intended for the peer-reviewed literature. Logdberg, for example, was once given responsibility for writing up case histories about a drug for subclinical hypothyroidism. The drug was approved by the FDA for hypothyroidism, but the company wanted physicians to prescribe it even when patients were not symptomatic. So the company convened a breakfast meeting with about fifteen physicians, who all knew one another and who were each paid for the meeting. "It was such a scam," says Logdberg. The physicians listened to the company presentation, and then the "first-adopters" talked about their great experiences prescribing the drug for subclinical hypothyroidism, all of which Logdberg wrote up. Her work was distributed to the company's drug reps, who used it to pitch the drug to doctors.

Part of the problem is that most agencies produce both scientific articles and marketing materials. And marketing, like politics and rhetoric, places a premium on the art of persuasion. Outright deception is forbidden, but shaping the facts to suit your message is an essential part of the game. Yet the concept of shaping the facts runs contrary to the internal ethos of science, which stipulates that numbers cannot be fiddled with and data cannot be cooked. If that ethos is disregarded, the entire scientific enterprise is shaken. "I had grown up in a scientific environment," says David Bronstein. "The very idea that you could bend the truth came as a huge shock." Yet in many agencies, both scientific articles and marketing articles are produced by the same writer. A medical writer who is composing supposedly objective review articles for a scientific journal about current therapies for schizophrenia will also be writing promotional materials for a manufacturer of a schizophrenia drug. "People I met in the industry all said they preferred the promotional aspect, because the medical education side is not only boring, they were uncomfortable with it," says Susan Gilbert. "With promotion, it was what it was." Gilbert worked at a medical communications agency for only five months before quitting. "I had a huge problem with doctors being educated by people like me and my colleagues, some of whom had PhDs, but many of which were just admen. These were people who worked at ad agencies and had that kind of mind-set."

When writers talk about medical communications agencies, a strange tone often creeps into their remarks. They seem to resent the ethos of marketing, and many of them look down on their business colleagues. But some medical writers also carry a heavy chip on their shoulders. Perhaps this is because so many of them still feel the sting of leaving behind a career in science. Or it may also be that all those years in universities insulated them from the most craven excesses of commerce. Still, listening to a writer talk about medical communications is often like listening to an earnest ex-hippie from Berkeley talk about a friend who betrayed peace and love for a career in investment banking. "These types of people—I was not even aware they existed," says David Bronstein. "Hard-faced, pushy people. Lots of women wearing power suits. Ghastly personalities. There are a lot more lizards in that company than in the general population."

The resentment may also simply be the consequence of the brutal, high-pressure working atmosphere of many agencies. Gilbert says, "I kid you not: there were people who would work through the night. A typical workday was, get in at eight or eight thirty and stay until nine." She says many of her fellow writers complained about getting burned out, yet that did not prevent them from putting in punishing hours. "The work is so useless, yet this is a twenty-four/seven business," says Gilbert. "There were colleagues of mine who worked through their Thanksgiving vacation."

Bronstein says that while the agency expected him to work long hours, it also tried to create a "work hard and play hard" atmosphere. *Enforced gaiety* is the term he uses to describe it. One year, about fifty employees were instructed to turn up at the agency with their passports. "They got us sozzled on white wine at eight a.m., and then flew us from the UK to Toronto for the weekend for helicopter flights around Niagara Falls and lots of frenetically scheduled partying," Bronstein recalls. He says that the company directors set the mandatory "fun all the way" tone in the middle of the transatlantic flight by starting a food fight with the British Airways meals. "It was bedlam," Bronstein says. As buns and drinks flew across the cabin of the plane, the flight attendants and other passengers watched in stunned disbelief. Bronstein says, "There was something about the vulgarity of it all, the disregard of other people, the cynicism and, of course, the greed of the entire trip that was precisely in accord with the culture of that company."

•   •   •

Scientific journals are sometimes seen as stalwarts of the honor-bound scholarly tradition, defenders of truth against spin. And it is certainly true that some of the most outspoken critics of the commercial imperative have been editors or ex-editors of the leading medical journals. Yet most medical journals have their own conflicts of interest. Journals are financed in part by advertising placed by pharmaceutical companies. In 2004, the American Medical Association generated 15.1 percent of its total revenue from advertisements in its journals, including *JAMA*. American Medical Association journals generated twice as much that year from advertising revenue ($40.7 million) as they did from subscriptions.[24]

Many people think of academic publishing as a dusty, somewhat threadbare endeavor. In fact, scientific publishing, unlike most academic publishing, is an extraordinarily profitable business. From 2000 to 2005, Reed Elsevier, the world's largest publisher of scientific journals, including the *Lancet*, earned profits of close to $10 billion.[25] Scientific journals used to be published by a broad range of groups—professional societies, university presses, nonprofit organizations, and academic publishing companies. But over the past two decades the field has come to be dominated by a handful of large multinational publishers. These publishers have a virtual stranglehold on university libraries, which must subscribe to scientific journals in order for faculty members to do their work. Many publishers have begun to bundle their journals together in electronic packages, often charging outlandish subscription fees. For a subscription to the *Journal of Comparative Neurology*, for instance, Wiley InterScience charges libraries $30,212 a year.[26] The Elsevier journal *Brain Research* comes with an annual price tag of $23,655.[27] Even a publication as obscure as Springer's *Lithuanian Mathematical Journal* costs $3,007 a year.[28]

Part of what makes such extraordinary fees possible is the fact that journal publishers do not have to pay contributors. In fact, the content of the journals is provided largely by the very academics whose institutions are paying such enormous subscription fees. Academic researchers submit their work for free to scientific journals, donate their time to peer-review the work of others, and sometimes even edit the journals without charge. Yet the high price of the journals often means that few people without a university appointment or corporate backing can afford the subscription fees. For instance, as things stand now, it is entirely possible that I might write an article on the University of Minnesota's dime, submit it to a journal to which I have also donated my time as a reviewer, sign over the copyright to the journal's publisher, and then ask my students to pay the publisher again to get copies of the article in my course-reading packet—all for a commercial publishing company that charges my university thousands of dollars annually in institutional subscription fees. It is this arrangement that has led Richard Smith, the former editor of the *British Medical Journal*, to write, "The whole business of medical journals is corrupt because owners are making money from restricting access to important research, most of it funded by public money."[29]

Journal editors sometimes claim that they block excessive industry influence by building firewalls between their marketing and editorial departments. If the marketing arm of the company is walled off from any contact with the editorial arm, the editors are supposedly insulated from making publication decisions based on commercial considerations. Yet these firewalls have not always prevented drug companies from playing hardball when their interests are challenged. For instance, in 1992, when a study in the *Annals of Internal Medicine* pointed out the inaccuracy of drug advertisements in medical journals, a number of pharmaceutical companies simply withdrew their advertising from the journal, costing the publication an estimated $1.5 million in lost revenue.[30] This kind of financial blowback is hard for an editor to ignore.

Drug advertisements are not the most problematic source of industry revenue for medical journals, however. When a pharmaceutical company publishes an article that reflects well on its drug, the company will often pay the journal large fees for reprints of the article, which drug reps for the company then distribute free of charge to doctors as a way of marketing the drug. These reprint fees are surprisingly high, especially in an age of electronic publication. They also present a conflict of interest that cannot be easily managed with firewalls, because an editor can often tell in advance which articles are likely to bring in big reprint fees (for instance, a large, positive clinical trial of a new drug). For example, the *New England Journal of Medicine* sold 929,400 reprints of Merck's VIGOR study, the notoriously misleading trial of Vioxx that Merck used as a major marketing tool. These reprints brought in between $697,000 and $836,000 for the *NEJM*.[31] The *NEJM* eventually repudiated the VIGOR study, but it did not return the money.

Some medical journals sell space to pharmaceutical companies in special journal supplements—sponsored issues usually devoted to a single topic. Often these supplements are the result of an industry-funded symposium, roundtable, or teleconference, where all the contributors have been recruited and paid by the sponsor and where the articles have been prepared by a ghostwriter. The *Journal of Clinical Psychiatry*, for instance, one of the most notorious supplement publishers, often produces more supplements in a single year than it does regular issues of the journal. In 2007, it published fourteen supplements on topics ranging from insomnia and atypical depression to ADHD and bipolar disorder in women. The articles in journal supplements are indexed in most library databases, and to all outward appearances, they look just like the peer-reviewed articles in the journal. By and large, however, sponsored articles are poorer in quality, not peer-reviewed, and more likely to be slanted toward the interests of the sponsor.[32]

Some journal publishers work even closer with industry. When Merck was promoting Vioxx in Australia, it contracted with a subsidiary of the scientific publisher Elsevier to produce a publication titled *Australasian Journal of Bone and Joint Medicine*. The publication looked much like a legitimate journal, complete with a masthead of prominent academic advisers. In fact, it was a marketing tool for Merck products. Of the twenty-nine articles in the second issue of the journal, nine were related to Vioxx, the anti-inflammatory drug that Merck was forced to withdraw from the market in 2004. Twelve were connected to Fosamax, an osteoporosis drug also produced by Merck. Unsurprisingly, the articles all reached positive conclusions about Merck products, and none disclosed the funding source. Excerpta Medica, the Elsevier-owned medical communications agency that produced the journal, also produced fake journals such as the *Australasian Journal of General Practice,* the *Australasian Journal of Neurology,* the *Australasian Journal of Cardiology,* the *Australasian Journal of Clinical Pharmacy,* and the *Australasian Journal of Cardiovascular Medicine.*[33]

• • •

Medical ghostwriting is not new. Neither is the use of scientific articles as marketing devices. What has changed is the sheer size and scope of the marketing enterprise. Over the past three decades, drug promotion has become a vast, complex bureaucratic machine, where strangers are connected to one another by a web of contracts, fees, and specialized agencies. Pharmaceutical companies have been joined by advertising companies, publishing companies, public relations firms, medical education agencies, and university CME offices, each with its own set of skills, services, and financial incentives. To understand how this network of financial relationships has changed medical communication, consider two promotional scandals separated by a period of thirty years.

On February 2, 1959, the pharmaceutical company Richardson-Merrell acquired the rights to market a new sedative in the United States.[34] The drug had been developed by a German firm that was selling it as an over-the-counter medication. In Sweden, it was marketed as the "babysitter" drug, a medication that frazzled mothers could use to sedate their children. Richardson-Merrell, however, did not plan to market the drug as a general sedative; they planned to market it as a treatment for the nausea of pregnancy. The drug was known in the United States by the trade name Kevadon, and in Germany by the name Contergan, but today it is better known by its generic name, thalidomide.

Today few people remember thalidomide as a sedative. They remember it as a toxic agent that caused thousands of severe, disabling birth defects. By the early 1960s, it was clear that an alarming number of women in Europe taking thalidomide for sedation or nausea were giving birth to children with phocomelia, or malformed, flipperlike arms and legs. About eight thousand children were born with gross deformities, and it is estimated that as many as seven thousand fetuses may have died before birth.[35] Although thalidomide was never actually marketed in the United States, Richardson-Merrell gave it to patients in clinical trials. One of these trials was reported in a ghostwritten journal article that declared the drug safe and effective for pregnant women.

Richardson-Merrell, the American distributor for thalidomide, was never a major drug producer. It was a subsidiary of the Vick Chemical Company, known mainly for producing cough drops and Vicks VapoRub. So when executives of Richardson-Merrell decided to market thalidomide as a treatment for nausea in pregnancy, they did not immediately think of conducting research to see if it was safe for fetuses. They thought first of recruiting a doctor to testify to its safety. When people at Richardson-Merrell proposed this idea to an editor at the *American Journal of Obstetrics and Gynecology,* the editor replied that before the company could declare thalidomide safe for fetuses, it would at least need to find out if the drug crossed the placental barrier. The company did not have this information.

Richardson-Merrell decided to test the drug in humans, but instead of actually designing research to see if the drug crossed the placental barrier, it carried out marketing trials—uncontrolled "studies" on unknowing patients, managed by the company's marketing department and designed to sell doctors and hospitals on the merits of thalidomide.[36] Richardson-Merrell sent out 2.5 million tablets of thalidomide to 1,267 doctors, who gave them to approximately 20,000 patients. The company told its drug reps to assure doctors that they "need not report results if they don't want to." As Richardson-Merrell was distributing thalidomide to patients, however, its animal studies began to show that rats given the drug died at an alarmingly high rate. Richardson-Merrell pressed on with human testing. When doctors began reporting side effects in their patients, especially peripheral nerve damage, the company redoubled its efforts to find something positive to publish.[37]

In 1961, the *American Journal of Obstetrics and Gynecology* published an article by Dr. Roy Nulsen testifying that thalidomide was safe, effective, and suitable as an antinausea drug for women in the late stages of pregnancy.[38] In fact, the article had been ghostwritten by the medical director of Richardson-Merrell, Dr. Raymond Pogge, with the help of his secretary. Roy Nulsen, the "author," was a Cincinnati physician who had taken part in the marketing trial of thalidomide. He had nothing to do with writing the article, however. Nulsen later confessed that he had not even kept track of how many pills he'd dispensed or which patients he had given them to. He also said that he had not actually communicated any data to Richardson-Merrell in writing but that he had talked on the telephone to Pogge, "or it may have been that we had lunch together, or it may have been when we played golf."[39]

In retrospect, what is striking about the thalidomide ghosting episode is how informal it was. Pogge wrote the article; Nulsen signed it. There were no middlemen involved—no medical writers, no publication planners, no medical education agencies. No complex bureaucracy stood between Pogge, the pharmaceutical company executive, and Nulsen, the local physician. They played golf together. In fact, by the standards of today, neither Richardson-Merrell nor the journal that published the ghosted article made much effort to pretend that the article was scientifically sound.

Compare, then, a similar scandal that took place thirty years later: the marketing of Fen-Phen, the notorious weight-loss drug produced by Wyeth. Fen-Phen was withdrawn from the market in 1997 after it was linked to valvular heart disease. By some estimates, valvular disease affected as many as 30 percent of the seven million Fen-Phen users.[40] Soon thereafter, Fen-Phen was also linked to primary pulmonary hypertension, an even deadlier disease. By 2001, Wyeth had acknowledged that at least 450,000 patients had become ill as a result of using the drug; at least 365,000 of those patients had joined a mass federal settlement. No uncontroversial figures exist as to how many Fen-Phen users died, but it is probably safe to say that at a minimum, they number in the hundreds.

As Alicia Mundy has documented in her book *Dispensing with the Truth,* the behavior of Wyeth officials during the safety crisis was not exactly a model of corporate responsibility. In 1997, clinicians in Fargo, North Dakota, and at the Mayo Clinic notified Wyeth that they had seen thirteen patients on Fen-Phen who had developed valvular disease. Wyeth responded by destroying the data. The Wyeth safety officer went to the files and "overwrote" them to them to avoid any mention of valvular disease.[41] Wyeth then sat on the information about valvular disease for several more months before notifying the FDA. Wyeth's approach to the worries about primary pulmonary hypertension was not much better. One company bureaucrat's memo that was unearthed in litigation read,

Can I look forward to my waning years signing checks for fat people who are a little afraid of some silly lung problem? [42]

From the very start, ghostwriting was a key piece of the Fen-Phen marketing plan. Unlike the thalidomide episode thirty years earlier, however, this was not an informal agreement between two golfing buddies. The ghostwritten Fen-Phen articles were the product of a complex multimillion-dollar public relations strategy. In 1996 Wyeth hired Excerpta Medica, Inc., a New Jersey-based medical communications firm, to write ten articles for medical journals promoting treatment for obesity. Wyeth paid Excerpta Medica $20,000 per article. In turn, Excerpta Medica paid prominent university researchers $1,000 to $1,500 to edit drafts of the articles and put their names on the published product. Excerpta Medica, a branch of the academic publisher Elsevier, manages two medical journals itself: *Clinical Therapeutics* and *Current Therapeutic Research*. According to court documents, Excerpta Medica planned to submit most of the articles it produced to Elsevier journals. In the actual event, Excerpta managed to publish only two articles before Fen-Phen was withdrawn from the market, in 1997. One appeared in *Clinical Therapeutics*, the other in the *American Journal of Medicine*, another Elsevier journal.

Wyeth kept each article under tight control, scrubbing drafts of any material with the potential to damage sales.[43] So clean was the laundering operation, in fact, that many of the authors did not even realize that Wyeth was involved. One of the authors, Richard Atkinson of the University of Wisconsin, sent a letter to Excerpta Medica congratulating them on the thoroughness and clarity of their article. "Perhaps I can get you to write all my papers for me!" he wrote. He did have one reservation about the article he was signing: "My only general comment is that this piece may make dexfenfluramine sound better than it really is."[44]

Wyeth's "medical education" campaign for Fen-Phen was a model of the modern genre. The campaign cast obesity as a dangerous public-health problem for which Fen-Phen was the remedy. The $54 million set aside by Wyeth to launch the drug included grants to the American Academy of Family Physicians, the American Diabetes Association, the North American Society for the Study of Obesity, and the American Society of Bariatric Physicians. Wyeth budgeted $700,000 for C. Everett Koop's advocacy group Shape Up America; $275,000 for a "State of Weight" teleseminar; $179,000 for "Dear Doctor" letters; and $50,000 for a women's health seminar.[45] Wyeth also maintained a stable of high-profile thought leaders, including JoAnn Manson of Harvard and Gerald Faich of the University of Pennsylvania, who together wrote a complimentary editorial on Fen-Phen for the *New England Journal of Medicine* (without disclosing their corporate ties), and George Blackburn, the chair of the Committee on Nutrition for the Massachusetts Medical Society, who was instrumental in getting Massachusetts to lift a ban on Fen-Phen.[46]

When evidence mounted showing that Fen-Phen was causing people to die, Wyeth did not back off. In fact, the company put its public relations machine into high gear. Even after Fen-Phen had been withdrawn from the market, Wyeth spent $100 million on public relations to convince people that that response had been overblown.[47] It convened an "expert panel" of cardiologists and gave Arthur Weyman of Harvard an honorarium of five thousand dollars a day to chair it.[48] It put together a Very Important Visiting Professor (VIVP) program and flew the VIVPs to CME events at exotic resorts.[49] Most critical, Wyeth funded studies to look for evidence that minimized the safety worries about Fen-Phen—and if the studies' results were favorable, the company publicized them heavily. For example, Wyeth spent over $18 million on a study by Neil Weissman at Georgetown University examining valvular damage. When a preliminary analysis of the unpublished data looked somewhat favorable, it was presented at a conference, promoted by press release, and featured on the front page of *USA Today* with the headline "Study: No Heart Damage from Diet Drug." (That analysis was later discredited.)[50]

In a way, the difference between the introduction of Fen-Phen in the mid-1990s and that of thalidomide in the early 1960s is emblematic of much larger changes in medicine itself. The period separating these two drugs was the era in which scientific medicine took root and became institutionalized. The individual clinical judgment of the physician was being replaced by larger mechanisms designed to enforce the conclusions of scientific evidence. The solo practitioner, with all his quirks and idiosyncrasies, was entering the complex world of randomized clinical trials, practice guidelines, consensus committees, rating scales, and evidence-based medicine. This world also introduced new pressure points for pharmaceutical companies. No longer was it sufficient for companies simply to exert influence over individual practitioners by sending out drug reps to distribute samples. They also needed to influence the larger structures that were assuming such importance.

The marketing of Fen-Phen reflected this shift. It was not enough for Wyeth to persuade doctors individually to prescribe Fen-Phen. The company also had to influence the various expert panels, consensus committees, advocacy groups, professional societies, medical education programs, and scientific journal articles that would determine how Fen-Phen was prescribed. Ghostwriting played a part, but it was only a small part of a much larger and more complex marketing plan. As doctors have begun to look more and more to science for their prescribing decisions, the marketing of prescription drugs has begun to look more and more like science.

．　．　．

When you look at some of the figures in the pharmaceutical marketing system, it is not hard to see the appeal of the industry's jobs. For the drug reps, there is the con-man challenge of pitting yourself against an unwitting doctor. For the thought leaders, there is the ego stroke of being treated like a celebrity. For the guinea pigs, there is the appeal of working off the grid. But what is there for the ghostwriters? There is good money, of course; the job does supply a decent living. And if you are a freelancer, you often get to work from home and set your own schedule. But the job itself does not sound like much fun, even if it is all on the up-and-up. Lots of data, lots of numbers, lots of hours logged in front of a computer screen, broken up by interludes with puffed-up academic physicians who get the credit for your work, all while taking orders from twenty-five-year-old account managers. It does not sound like the most rewarding way to spend a life. "Ethically dubious and soul-crushingly dull" is the way one disillusioned ex-writer put it. Even the well-intentioned writers struggle when they try to explain why they enjoy the job.

"Well, it sounds dumb, but I like writing down what other people say," says Linda Logdberg. "I like taking notes and trying accurately to represent what's happened." Before she became a writer, Logdberg was on track for a successful academic career. She had published two articles in *Science*, a significant benchmark of academic success. But Logdberg felt that academic life was too sedentary, required too many committee meetings, and involved too much quibbling and pontificating by hyper-confident scientists. "I looked at most of the alphas and neither identified with nor liked them," she says. Medical writing satisfied her intellectual curiosity and allowed her to avoid the academic pressure cooker created by the tenure clock. Medical writing did not even seem ethically troubling at first. It only began to seem corrupt during the mid- to late 1990s when she was working for firms owned by advertising companies. Then her irritation began to kick in. Logdberg says, "I found myself working for advertising chickies who were wearing those wasp-waisted black suits and were eternally twenty-six years old."

One warm fall night last year, I drove across town to St. Paul for a meeting of the local chapter of the American Medical Writers Association. It was a small affair, held over dinner at the student union of the University of St. Thomas, and the topic for the evening was ethics. Sitting to my right at the table was a pleasant woman who told me she managed a market research company that was looking for medical writers. On my left was a middle-aged man with graying hair and an open-collared shirt. When I asked him what brought him to the meeting, he said, "Desperation." He explained that he used to be a nurse but had lost his license. He had been out of work for four months, and he thought he might start over as a medical writer.

I had gone to the meeting expecting fireworks. At most medical meetings, few issues are more likely to generate hard feelings than a debate about ethics and the pharmaceutical industry. And after a series of high-profile revelations about industry ghostwriting, I had the impression that medical writers were defensive and more than a little worried about their future. The ethics of ghostwriting had been a hot issue on AMWA listservs, as well as in its in-house publication and at its annual conference. But the evening at St. Thomas was a surprisingly sedate affair. There was quiet conversation over lasagna and tossed salad, followed by a couple of bland lectures on the ethics of medical writing. No one got angry. No sharp words were exchanged. The writers around the table didn't seem craven, or greedy, or even especially defensive. I saw no power suits or expensive shoes. The dinner seemed like a staff gathering for a human resources department whose employees were all middle-aged women.

Perhaps I should not have been surprised. It is not as if medical writers are high-powered decision-makers. They are well-paid technicians who perform a specialized service for their clients, often without a whole lot of agonizing about the ethics. This attitude is understandable. Even if writers were to cultivate a little moral anguish, they probably could not do a lot with it. Their moral problem is not simply that their jobs occasionally stray into unethical territory. The problem lies in the structure of the job itself. Like lobbyists, expert witnesses, or hit men, medical writers are instruments in a much larger enterprise. Their job is neither to support nor question the enterprise, but to play their small part as effectively as possible.

A few years ago David Bronstein went to a major cardiology congress in Barcelona, organized by a friend in the business. One evening Bronstein had dinner with a group of medical writers. They were a friendly bunch, and like-minded, but he found them terribly sad. "Over time, ghostwriters start to resemble ghosts," he says. "They come to look faded, run-down, and sort of worm-blown." Whether it is owing to the moral compromises or the petty humiliations, Bronstein does not say. Medical writing has little glamour, and whatever moral purpose it might once have carried has been rubbed away by the constant friction with commerce. The fact that writing is such hard work just makes it worse. If you are a true believer in the glory of the market, the work might be invigorating, and the long hours a mark of pride. But if you are a lapsed biologist, raised in the church of science but forced to leave, it is a source of nagging bitterness and resentment. Ghostwriting pays the mortgage, but it wears at the soul. Bronstein says, "What a wretched epitaph to a life this would be."

CHAPTER THREE

The Detail Men

BACK IN THE OLD DAYS, long before drug companies started making headlines in the business pages, doctors were routinely called upon by company representatives known as detail men. To "detail" a doctor is to give that doctor information about a company's new drugs with the aim of persuading the doctor to prescribe them. When I was growing up, in South Carolina in the 1970s, I would occasionally see detail men sitting patiently in the waiting room outside the office of my father, a family doctor. They were pretty easy to spot. Detail men were usually sober, conservatively dressed gentlemen who would not have looked out of place at the Presbyterian church across the street. Instead of Bibles or hymn books, though, they carried detail bags, which were filled with journal articles, drug samples, and branded knickknacks for the office.

Today detail men are officially known as pharmaceutical sales representatives, but everyone I know calls them drug reps. Drug reps are still easy to spot in a clinic or hospital, but for slightly different reasons than in the past. The most obvious is their appearance. It is probably fair to say that doctors, pharmacists, and medical-school professors are not generally admired for their good looks and fashion sense. Against this backdrop, the average drug rep looks like a supermodel, or maybe an A-list movie star. Drug reps today are often young, well groomed, and strikingly good-looking. Many are women. They are usually affable and sometimes very smart. Many give off a kind of glow, as if they have just emerged from a spa or salon. And they are always, hands down, the best-dressed people in the hospital.

Drug reps have been calling on doctors since the mid-nineteenth century, but during the late 1990s their numbers increased dramatically. From 1996 to 2001 the pharmaceutical sales force in America doubled, to a total of 90,000 reps.[1] By 2005, there was a drug rep for every 2.5 doctors in America.[2] One reason is simple: good reps move product. Detailing is expensive, but almost all practicing doctors see reps at least occasionally, and many doctors say they find reps useful. One study found that for drugs introduced after 1997 with revenues exceeding $200 million a year, the average return for each dollar spent on detailing was $10.29.[3] That is an impressive figure. It is almost twice the return on investment in medical-journal advertising, and more than seven times the return on direct-to-consumer advertising.

But the relationship between doctors and drug reps has never been uncomplicated, for reasons that should be obvious. The first duty of doctors, at least in theory, is to their patients. Doctors must make prescribing decisions based on medical evidence and their own clinical judgments. Drug reps, in contrast, are salespeople. They swear no oaths, take care of no patients, and profess no high-minded ethical duties. Their job is to persuade doctors to prescribe their drugs. If reps are lucky, their drugs are good, the studies are clear, and their job is easy. But sometimes reps must persuade doctors to prescribe drugs that are marginally effective, exorbitantly expensive, difficult to administer, or even dangerously toxic. Reps that succeed are rewarded with bonuses or commissions. Reps that fail may find themselves unemployed.

Most people who work in health care, if they give drug reps any thought at all, regard them with mixed feelings. A handful avoid reps as if they were vampires, backing out of the room when they see one approaching. In their view, the best that can be said about reps is that they are a necessary by-product of a market economy. They view reps much as NBA players used to view Michael Jordan: as an awesome, powerful force that you can never really stop, only hope to control.

Yet many reps are so friendly, so easygoing, so much fun to flirt with that it is virtually impossible to demonize them. How can you demonize someone who brings you lunch and touches your arm and remembers your birthday and knows the names of all your children? After a while even the most steel-willed doctors may look forward to visits by a rep, if only in the self-interested way that they look forward to the UPS truck pulling up in the driveway. A rep at the door means a delivery has arrived: takeout for the staff, trinkets for the kids, and, most indispensable, drug samples on the house. Although samples are the single largest marketing expense for the drug industry, they pay handsome dividends:

doctors who accept samples of a drug are far more likely to prescribe that drug later on than doctors who don't.

Drug reps may well have more influence on prescriptions than anyone in America other than doctors themselves, but to most people outside the drug industry their jobs are mysterious. What exactly do they do every day? Where do they get their information? What do they say about doctors when the doctors are not around? Reps can be found in hospitals, waiting rooms, and conference halls all over the country, yet they barely register on the collective medical consciousness. Many doctors notice them only in the casual, utilitarian way that one might notice a waitress or a bartender. Some doctors look down on them on ethical grounds. "Little Willy Lomans," they say, "only in it for the money." When I asked my friends and colleagues in medicine to suggest some reps I could talk to about detailing, most could not come up with a single name.

These doctors may be right about reps. It is true that selling pharmaceuticals can be a highly lucrative job. But in a market-based medical system, are reps really so different from doctors? Most doctors in the United States now work, directly or indirectly, for large corporations. Like reps, many doctors must answer to managers and bureaucrats. They are overwhelmed by paperwork and red tape. Unlike my father, who would sooner have walked to Charleston barefoot than take out an ad for his practice, many doctors now tout their services on roadside billboards. My medical-school alumni magazine recently featured the Class of 1988 valedictorian, who has written a diet book, started her own consulting firm, and become the national spokesperson for a restaurant chain. For better or worse, America has turned its health-care system over to the same market forces that transformed the village hardware store into a Home Depot and the corner pharmacy into a strip-mall CVS. Its doctors are moving to the same medical suburb where drug reps have lived for the past hundred and fifty years. If they want to know what life in the suburbs is like, perhaps they should talk to the people who live there.

•   •   •

Gene Carbona was almost a criminal. I know this because thirty minutes into our first telephone conversation, he told me, "Carl, I was almost a criminal." I have heard ex–drug reps speak bluntly about their former jobs, but never quite so cheerfully and openly. These days Carbona works for the *Medical Letter,* a highly respected nonprofit publication, but he was telling me about his twelve years working for Merck and then Astra Merck, a firm initially set up to market the Sweden-based Astra's drugs in the United States (Carbona stresses that he is speaking only for himself).[4] Carbona began training as a rep in 1988, when he was only eleven days out of college. He detailed two drugs for Astra Merck. One was a calcium-channel blocker he calls "a dog." The other was the heartburn medication Prilosec, which at the time was available by prescription only.

Prilosec is the kind of drug most reps can only dream about. The industry considers a drug to be a blockbuster if it reaches a billion dollars a year in sales. In 1998 Prilosec became the first drug in America to reach $5 billion a year.[5] In 2000 it made $6 billion.[6] Prilosec's success was not the result of a massive heartburn epidemic. It was based on the same principle that drove the success of many other 1990s blockbusters, from Vioxx to Viagra: the restoration of an ordinary biological function that time and circumstance had eroded. In the case of Prilosec, the function was digestion. Many people discovered that the drug allowed them to eat the burritos and curries that their gastrointestinal systems had placed off-limits. So what if Prilosec was four dollars a pill, as compared to a quarter or so for a Tagamet? Patients still begged for it. Prilosec was their savior. Astra Merck marketed Prilosec as the "purple pill," but according to Carbona, many patients called it "purple Jesus."

How did Astra Merck do it? Prilosec was the first proton-pump inhibitor (a drug that inhibits the production of stomach acid) approved by the Food and Drug Administration, and thus the first drug available in its class. By definition this gave it a considerable head start on the competition. In the late 1990s Astra Merck mounted a huge direct-to-consumer campaign; ads for the purple pill were ubiquitous. But consumer advertising can do only so much for a drug because doctors, not patients, write the prescriptions. This is where reps become indispensable.

Many reps can tell stories about occasions when, in order to move their product, they pushed the envelope of what is ethically permissible. I have heard reps talk about scoring sports tickets for their favorite doctors, buying televisions for waiting rooms, and arranging junkets to tropical resorts. One rep told me he set up a putting green in a hospital and gave a putter to any doctor who made a hole in one. A former rep told me about a colleague who somehow managed to persuade a pharmacist to let him secretly write the prescribing protocol for antibiotic use at a local hospital and then put his company's product as the first choice for many patients.

But Carbona was in a class of his own. He had access to so much money for doctors that he had trouble spending it all. He took residents out to bars. He distributed "unrestricted educational grants." He arranged to buy lunch for the staff of certain private practices every day for a year. Often he would invite a group of doctors and their guests to a high-end restaurant, buy them drinks and a lavish meal, open up the club in back, and party until 4:00 a.m. "The more money I spent," Carbona says, "the more money I made." If he came back to the restaurant later that week with his wife, everything would be on the house. "My money was no good at restaurants," he told me, "because I was the King of Happy Hour."

My favorite Carbona story, the one that left me shaking my head in admiration, took place in Tallahassee. One of the more important clinics Carbona called on was a practice there consisting of about fifty doctors. Although the practice had plenty of patients, it was struggling. This problem was not uncommon. When the movement toward corporate-style medicine got under way, in the 1980s and 1990s, many doctors found themselves ill-equipped to run a business; they didn't know much about how to actually make money. ("That's why doctors are such great targets for Ponzi schemes and real-estate scams," Carbona helpfully points out.) Carbona was detailing this practice twice a week and had gotten to know some of the clinicians pretty well. At one point a group of them asked him for help. " 'Gene, you work for a successful business,'" Carbona recalls them saying. " 'Is there any advice you could give us to help us turn the practice around?' " At this point he knew he had stumbled upon an extraordinary opportunity.

Carbona decided that the clinic needed a "practice-management consultant." And he and his colleagues at Astra Merck knew just the man: a financial planner and accountant with whom they were very friendly. They wrote up a contract. They agreed to pay the consultant a flat fee of about $50,000 to advise the clinic. But they also gave him another incentive. Carbona says, "We told him that if he was successful there would be more business for him in the future, and by *successful*, we meant a rise in prescriptions for our drugs."

The consultant did an extremely thorough job. He spent eleven or twelve hours a day at the clinic for months. He talked to every employee, from the secretaries to the nurses to the doctors. He thought carefully about every aspect of the practice, from the most mundane administrative details to big-picture matters such as bill collection and financial strategy. He turned the practice into a profitable, smoothly running financial machine. And prescriptions for Astra Merck drugs soared.

When I asked Carbona how the consultant had increased Astra Merck's market share within the clinic so dramatically, he said that the consultant never pressed the doctors directly. Instead, he talked up Carbona. "Gene has put his neck on the line for you guys," he would tell them. "If this thing doesn't work, he might get fired." The consultant emphasized what a remarkable service the practice was getting, how valuable the financial advice was, how everything was going to turn around for them—all courtesy of Carbona. The strategy worked. "Those guys went berserk for me," Carbona says. Doctors at the newly vitalized practice prescribed so many Astra Merck drugs that he got a $140,000 bonus. The scheme was so successful that Carbona and his colleagues at Astra Merck decided to duplicate it in other practices.

I got in touch with Carbona after I learned that he was giving talks on the American Medical Student Association lecture circuit about his experiences as a rep. At that point I had read a fair bit of pharmaceutical sales literature, and most of it had struck me as remarkably hokey and stilted. Merck's official training materials, for example, instruct reps to say things like "Doctor, based on the information we discussed today, will you prescribe Vioxx for your patients who need once-daily power to prevent pain due to osteoarthritis?" So I was unprepared for a man with Carbona's charisma and forthright humor. I could see why he had been such an excellent rep: he came off as a cross between a genial con artist and a comedic character actor. After two hours on the phone with him I probably would have bought anything he was selling.

Most media accounts of the pharmaceutical industry miss this side of drug reps. By focusing on scandals—the kickbacks and the fraud and the lavish gifts—they lose sight of the fact that many reps are genuinely likable people. The better ones have little use for the canned scripts they are taught in training. For them, effective selling is all about developing a relationship with a doctor. If a doctor likes a rep, that doctor is going to feel bad about refusing to see the rep, or about taking his lunches and samples but never prescribing his drugs. As Jordan Katz, a rep for Schering-Plough until recently, says, "A lot of doctors just write for who they like."

A variation on this idea emerges in *Side Effects*, Kathleen Slattery-Moschkau's 2005 film about a fictional fledgling drug rep. Slattery-Moschkau, who worked for nine years as a rep for Bristol-Myers Squibb and Johnson and Johnson, says the carefully rehearsed messages in the corporate training courses really got to her. "I hated the crap I had to say to doctors," she told me. The heroine of *Side Effects* eventually decides to ditch the canned messages and stop spinning her product. Instead, she is brutally honest. "Bottom line?" she says to one doctor. "Your patients won't shit for a week." To her amazement, she finds that the blunter she is, the higher her market share rises. Soon she is winning sales awards and driving a company BMW.

For most reps, market share is the yardstick of success. The more scripts their doctors write for their drugs, the more the reps make. Slattery-Moschkau says that most of her fellow reps made $50,000 to $90,000 a year in salary and another $30,000 to $50,000 in bonuses, depending on how much they sold. Reps are pressured to "make quota," or meet yearly sales targets, which often increase from year to year. Reps who fail to make quota must endure the indignity of having their district manager frequently accompany them on sales calls. Those who meet quota are rewarded handsomely. The most successful reps achieve minor celebrity within the company.

One perennial problem for reps is the doctor who simply refuses to see them at all. Reps call these doctors No Sees. Cracking a No See is a genuine achievement, the pharmaceutical equivalent of a home run or a windmill dunk. Gene Carbona says that when he came across a No See, or any other doctor who was hard to influence, he used Northeast-Southwest tactics. If you can't get to a doctor, he explains, you go after the people surrounding that doctor, showering them with gifts. Carbona might help support a Little League baseball team or a bowling league. After a while, the doctor would think, *Gene is doing such nice things for all these people, the least I can do is give him ten minutes of my time.* At that point, Carbona says, the sale was as good as made. "If you could get ten minutes with a doctor, your market share would go through the roof."

For decades the medical community has debated whether gifts and perks from reps have any real effect. Doctors insist that they do not. Studies in the medical literature indicate just the opposite.[7] The pharmaceutical industry has managed this debate skillfully, pouring vast resources into gifts for doctors while simultaneously reassuring them that their integrity prevents them from being influenced. For example, in an editorial in the journal *Health Affairs*, Bert Spilker, a vice president for PhRMA, the pharmaceutical trade group, defended the practice of gift-giving against critics who, he scornfully wrote, "fear that physicians are so weak and lacking in integrity that they would 'sell their souls' for a pack of M&M candies and a few sandwiches and doughnuts."[8]

One of the most novel studies of industry influence was conducted nearly two decades ago in Cleveland.[9] In the late 1980s, drug manufacturers had treated members of the Department of Internal Medicine at the Cleveland Clinic to a number of free trips to popular vacation spots under the guise of medical education. Two researchers at the Cleveland Clinic, James Orlowski and Leon Wateska, wanted to see if the free trips actually had any effect on physicians. To do this, the researchers picked two drugs, one an antibiotic and one a heart medicine, each made by a different manufacturer that had recently sponsored a free trip for the department. Then they reviewed the prescriptions written at their hospital for each drug. (Orlowski and Wateska had chosen medications that were only administered intravenously and so could easily be tracked through records at the hospital pharmacy.) First they looked at the use of the drugs during the twenty-two months before the department members were treated to an industry-funded trip, and then they looked at the seventeen months after the trip.

The change was astonishing. For the antibiotic, prescriptions during the period right after the trip spiked to *ten times* what they had been before the trip. Shortly thereafter prescriptions leveled off, but still they leveled off at a rate that was over three times higher than before the trip. For the heart drug, the jump was more modest, but it was still impressive: prescriptions increased to two and a half times what they'd been before the trip. In fact, prescriptions increased even before department members actually took the trip. Their first spike came immediately after the invitations were offered.

Over the past twenty years, the evidence that gifts and payments have a profound influence on doctors has become virtually indisputable. Doctors who are paid by a company are more likely to write prescriptions for that company's drugs, more likely to give talks that are favorable to the company, and more likely to produce research that benefits the company.[10] Even modest gifts have a substantial effect. A group at Case Western Reserve University tracked doctors' requests to have particular drugs added to the hospital formulary.[11] They found that the more industry ties a doctor had, the more likely that doctor was to request specific additions to the formulary. In fact, doctors who often accepted money for speaking engagements were almost thirty times more likely to ask for a specific drug to be added to the formulary than doctors who didn't.

For years, doctors have resisted the evidence that gifts affect their decisions. As Richard Waltman, a Washington family physician, writes, "I never compromised the health of a patient because of a free laser pointer or tennis balls."[12] Most doctors would agree. In the Cleveland Clinic study, almost all the doctors who took trips—nineteen of the twenty—had previously predicted that the trip was unlikely to influence their prescribing. In fact, according to one small study of medical residents in the *Canadian Medical Association Journal,* one way to convince a doctor that he or she cannot be influenced by gifts may be to give one; the more gifts a doctor takes, the more likely that doctor is to believe that the gifts have had no effect.[13] Even small gifts help. The gift itself may have no influence, but it might make a doctor more likely to think that he or she would not be influenced by larger gifts in the future. A pizza and a penlight are like inoculations, tiny injections of self-confidence that make a doctor think, *I will never be corrupted by money.*

These small gifts are ubiquitous. On a recent trip to South Carolina I started counting the drug company items that I could see in my parents' kitchen. On the refrigerator were magnets bearing the names Percocet, Relafen, Voltaren, Ultram, Prevacid, Mobic, Zomig-ZMT, Glynase, Aldomet, Exforge, Avandia, and Augmentin. A Coreg dish towel sat on the counter. Above the sink were bottles of lotion (Avelox) and hand gel (Tamiflu). When I looked down at the pen I was writing with, I saw the label *NuLev.* In a drawer were additional pens branded Zoloft, Zithromax, Truvada, Lipitor, Aciphex, Nexium, and Celexa. Upstairs in my bedroom closet I found tote bags bearing logos for Advair, Cipro, Imitrex, MetroGel Vaginal, Floxin, Procrit, Sanofi-Synthelabo, Schering, Aventis, Lyrica, Detrol LA. On the counter in the utility room was an item I at first thought was an obstetrics DVD but which on second glance turned out to be an instructional aid for Sunday school titled *A Clear View of the Birth of Jesus.*

Gifts from the drug industry are nothing new, of course. William Helfand, who worked in marketing for Merck for thirty-three years, told me that company representatives were giving doctors books and pamphlets as early as the late nineteenth century. "There is nothing new under the sun," Helfand says. "There is just more of it." The question is: Why is there so much more of it now? And what changed during the past two decades to bring about such a dramatic increase in reps bearing gifts?

•　•　•

One morning a few years ago I had breakfast at the Bryant-Lake Bowl, a diner in Minneapolis, with a former Pfizer rep named Michael Oldani. Oldani grew up in a working-class family in Kenosha, Wisconsin. Although he studied biochemistry in college, he knew nothing about pharmaceutical sales until he was recruited for Pfizer by the husband of a woman with whom he worked. Pfizer gave him a good salary, a company car, free gas, and an expense account. "It was kind of like the Mafia," Oldani told me. "They made me an offer I couldn't refuse." At the time, he was still in college and living with his parents. "I knew a good ticket out of Kenosha when I saw one," he said. He carried the bag for Pfizer for nine years, until 1998.

Today Oldani is a Princeton-trained medical anthropologist teaching at the University of Wisconsin at Whitewater. He wrote his doctoral dissertation on the anthropology of pharmaceutical sales, drawing not just on ethnographic fieldwork he did in Manitoba as a Fulbright scholar but also on his own experience as a rep. This dual perspective—the view of both a detached outsider and a street-savvy insider—gives his work authority and a critical edge. I had invited Oldani to lecture at the medical school of the University of Minnesota after reading his work in anthropology journals. Although his writing is scholarly, his manner is modest and self-effacing, more Kenosha than Princeton. This is a man who has spent a lot of time in diners.

Like Carbona, Oldani worked as a rep in the late 1980s and the 1990s, a period when the drug industry was undergoing key transformations. Its ethos was changing from that of the country-club establishment to the aggressive, new-money entrepreneur. Impressed by the success of AIDS activists in pushing for faster drug approvals, the drug industry increased pressure on the FDA to let companies bring drugs to the market more quickly. As a result, in 1992 Congress passed the Prescription Drug User Fee Act, under which drug companies pay a variety of fees to the FDA with the aim of speeding up drug approval (thereby making the drug industry a major funder of the agency set up to regulate it). In 1997 the FDA dropped most restrictions on direct-to-consumer advertising of prescription drugs, opening the gate for the eventual Levitra ads on Super Bowl Sunday and Zoloft cartoons during daytime television shows. The drug industry also became a big political player in Washington: by 2005, according to the Center for Public Integrity, its lobbying organization had become the largest in the country.[14]

Many companies started hitting for the fences, concentrating on potential blockbuster drugs for chronic illnesses in huge populations: Claritin for allergies, Viagra for impotence, Vioxx for arthritis, Prozac for depression. Successful drugs were followed by a flurry of competing me-too drugs. For most of the 1990s and the early part of the following decade, the pharmaceutical industry was easily the most profitable business sector in America. In 2002, according to Public Citizen, a nonprofit watchdog group, the combined profits of the top ten pharmaceutical companies in the Fortune 500 exceeded the combined profits of the other 490 companies.[15]

During this period, reps began to feel the influence of a new generation of executives intent on bringing market values to an industry that had been slow to embrace them. Anthony Wild, who was hired to lead Parke-Davis in the mid-1990s, told the journalist Greg Critser, the author of *Generation Rx*, that one of his first moves upon his appointment was to increase the incentive pay given to successful reps. Wild saw no reason to cap reps' incentives. As he said to the company's older executives, "Why not let them get rich?" Wild told the reps about the change at a meeting in San Francisco. "We announced that we were taking off the caps," he told Critser, "and the sales force went nuts!"[16]

It was not just the industry's ethos that was changing; the technology was changing too. According to Oldani, one of the most critical changes came in the way that information was gathered. In the days before computers, reps had to do a lot of legwork to figure out whom they could influence. They had to schmooze with the receptionists, make friends with the nurses, and chat up the pharmacists in order to learn which drugs the local doctors were prescribing, using the right incentives to coax what they needed from these informants. "Pharmacists are like pigeons," Jamie Reidy, a former rep for Pfizer and Eli Lilly, told me. "Only instead of bread crumbs, you toss them pizzas and sticky notes."

But in the 1990s, new information technology made it much simpler to track prescriptions. Market-research firms began collecting script-related data from pharmacies and hospitals and selling it to pharmaceutical companies.[17] The American Medical Association collaborated by licensing them information about doctors (including doctors who do not belong to the AMA), which it collects in its Physician Masterfile. Soon reps could find out exactly how many prescriptions any doctor was writing and exactly which drugs those prescriptions were for. All they had to do was turn on their laptops and download the data.

What they discovered was revelatory. For one thing, they found that a lot of doctors were lying to them. Doctors might tell a rep that they were writing prescriptions for, say, Lipitor, when they weren't. They were just being polite, or saying whatever they thought would get the rep off their backs. Now reps could detect the deception immediately. (Even today many doctors do not realize that reps have access to script-tracking reports.)

More important, prescription tracking helped reps figure out which doctors to target. They no longer had to waste time and money on doctors with conservative prescribing habits; they could head straight to the high prescribers, or high writers. The script-tracking report might even be accompanied by a profile of a physician put together by reps. (Oldani says, "A profile would be: 'Husband, three kids, loves needlepoint, off on Wednesdays. Amiable/expressive, brought up suicidality four times. High writer of Prozac. Won't accept tickets. Nurse says loves red wine, only French.'") Reps could get direct feedback on which tactics were working. If a gift or a dinner presentation did not result in more scripts, they knew to try another approach.

But there was the rub: the data was available to every rep from every company. The result was an arms race of pharmaceutical gift-giving, in which reps were forced to devise ever-new ways to exert influence. If the Eli Lilly rep was bringing sandwiches to the office staff, you brought Thai food. If GSK flew doctors to Palm Springs for a conference, you flew them to Paris. Oldani used to take residents to Major League Baseball games. "We did beer bongs, shots, and really partied," he told me. "Some of the guys were incredibly drunk on numerous occasions. I used to buy half barrels for their parties, almost on a retainer-like basis. I never talked product once to any of these residents, and they took care of me in their day-to-day practice. I never missed quota at their hospital."

Oldani says that script-tracking data also changed the way that reps thought about prescriptions. The old system of monitoring prescriptions was very inexact, and the relationship between a particular doctor's pre- scriptions and the work of a given rep was relatively hard to measure. But with precise script-tracking reports, reps started to feel a sense of ownership about prescriptions. If their doctors started writing more prescriptions for their drugs, the credit clearly belonged to the reps. However, more precise monitoring also invited micromanagement by the reps' bosses. They began pressuring reps to concentrate on high pre- scribers, fill out more paperwork, and report back to management more frequently.

"Script tracking, to me at least, made everyone a potentially success- ful rep," Oldani says. Reps didn't need to be nearly as resourceful and street-savvy as in the past; they just needed the script-tracking reports. The industry began hiring more and more reps, many with backgrounds in sales (rather than in, say, pharmacy, nursing, or biology). Some older reps say that during this period the industry replaced the serious detail man with "Pharma Barbie" and "Pharma Ken," whose medical knowl- edge was exceeded by their looks and catering skills. A newer, regimented style of selling began to replace the improvisational, more personal style of the old-school reps. Whatever was left of an ethic of service gave way to an ethic of salesmanship.

Doctors were caught in a bind. Many found themselves being called on several times a week by different reps from the same company. Most continued to see reps, some because they felt obligated to get up to speed with new drugs, some because they wanted to keep the pipeline of free samples open. But seeing reps has a cost, of course: the more reps a doctor sees, the longer the patients sit in the waiting room. Many doctors began to feel as though they deserved whatever gifts and perks they got because reps were such an irritation. At one time a few practices even charged reps a fee for visiting.

Professional organizations made some efforts to place limits on the gifts doctors were allowed to accept. These efforts were halfhearted, however, and they met with opposition from indignant doctors ridiculing the idea that their judgment could be bought. One doctor wrote a letter to the *American Medical News* confessing, "Every time a discussion comes up on guidelines for pharmaceutical company gifts to physicians, I feel as if I need to take a blood pressure medicine to keep from having a stroke."[18] In 2001 the AMA launched a campaign to educate doctors about the ethical perils of pharmaceutical gifts, but it undercut its message by funding the campaign with money from the pharmaceutical industry.

Of course, most doctors are never offered free trips to Monaco or even a weekend at a spa; for them an industry gift means a Cialis pen or a Lexapro notepad. Yet it is a rare rep who cannot tell a story or two about the extravagant gifts doctors have requested. Oldani told me that one doctor asked him to build a music room in his house. Phyllis Adams, a former rep in Canada, was told by a doctor that he would not prescribe her product unless her company made him a consultant. (Both said no.) Carbona arranged a $35,000 "unrestricted educational grant" for a doctor who wanted a swimming pool in his backyard. "It was the Wild West," says Jamie Reidy, whose frank memoir about his activities while working for Pfizer in the 1990s, *Hard Sell: The Evolution of a Viagra Salesman*, recently got him fired from Eli Lilly.[19] "They cashed the check, and that was it. And hopefully they remembered you every time they turned on the TV, or bought a drink on the cruise, or dived into the pool."

The trick is to give doctors gifts without making them feel that they are being bought. "Bribes that aren't considered bribes," Oldani says. "This, my friend, is the essence of pharmaceutical gifting." According to Oldani, the way to make a gift feel different from a bribe is to make it personal. "Ideally, a rep finds a way to get into a script writer's psyche," he says. "You need to have talked enough with a script writer—or done enough recon with gatekeepers—that you know what to give." When

Oldani found a pharmacist who liked to play the market, he gave him stock options. When he wanted to see a resistant oncologist, he talked to the doctor's nurse and then gave the oncologist a hundred-dollar bottle of his favorite cognac. Reidy put the point nicely when he told me, "You are absolutely buying love."

Such gifts do not come with an explicit quid pro quo, of course. Whatever obligation doctors feel to write scripts for a rep's products usually comes from the general sense of reciprocity implied by the ritual of gift-giving. (As the anthropologist Marcel Mauss asked in his classic book *The Gift*, "What power resides in the object that causes its recipient to pay it back?")[20] But it is impossible to avoid the hard reality informing these ritualized exchanges: reps would not give doctors free stuff if they did not expect more scripts.

My brother Hal, a psychiatrist currently on the faculty of Wake Forest University, told me about an encounter he had with a drug rep from Eli Lilly some years back, when he was in private practice. This rep was not one of his favorites; she was too aggressive. That day she had insisted on bringing lunch to his office staff, even though Hal had asked her not to. As he tried to make polite conversation with her in the hall, she reached over his shoulder into his drug closet and picked up a couple of sample packages of Zoloft and Celexa. Waving them in the air, she asked, "Tell me, Doctor, do the Pfizer and Forest reps bring lunch to your office staff?" A stony silence followed. Hal quietly ordered the rep out of the office and told her to never come back. She left in tears.

It's not hard to understand why Hal got so angry. The rep had broken the rules. Like an abrasive tourist who has not caught on to the code of manners in a foreign country, she had said outright the one thing that, by custom and common agreement, should never be said: the lunches she brought were intended as a bribe. What's more, they were a bribe that Hal had never agreed to accept. He likened the situation to having somebody drop off a bag of money in your garage without your consent and then ask, "So what about our little agreement?"

When an encounter between a doctor and a rep goes well, it is a delicate ritual of pretense and self-deception. Drug reps pretend that they are giving doctors impartial information. Doctors pretend that they take it seriously. Drug reps must try their best to influence doctors, while doctors must tell themselves that they are not being influenced. Drug reps must act as if they are not salespeople, while doctors must act as if they are not customers. And if, by accident, the real purpose of the exchange is revealed, the result is like an elaborate theatrical dance in which the masks and costumes suddenly drop off and the actors come face to face with one another as they really are. Nobody wants to see that happen.

•   •   •

Michael Oldani is telling me about his first job interview with Pfizer, back when he was still in college. "The regional sales manager asked me why I thought I'd be a good salesman, and I couldn't answer it," he says. "I had no idea what he was talking about." Then the manager saw that Oldani was carrying a black plastic portfolio. So he issued Oldani a challenge. "Sell me your portfolio," he said. Oldani replied, "Hey, how'd you like to buy this portfolio?" "I don't *need* that portfolio," said the manager, "I've got this leather one." Oldani shot back, "Yeah, well, this one's *plastic*. You can spill coffee on it and who cares? Make it your everyday one." The manager beamed. He had found a natural.

It is not a stretch to picture Oldani as a rep. Not as a pushy, jaded salesman or a hard-nosed closer, but more like the friendly, stand-up guy that you do your local business with—the waiter you joke around with at your neighborhood breakfast joint or the fellow behind the counter at the hardware store. It is easy to imagine him striding into an office with an armload of doughnuts to cries of "Hey, it's Mike!" like Norm walking into the bar on *Cheers*. A little harder to picture is how Oldani justified his job to himself, especially given his attitude toward the business a decade after leaving it. A genuine, decent sort, if not exactly a Boy Scout, Oldani did a lot of things as a rep that he now seems to regret. Yet at the time, he saw his tactics as well within the bounds of normal behavior—not exactly admirable, perhaps, but certainly not unforgivable sins. What was different back then?

Most companies get their rookie reps up to speed by sending them off for intense educational sessions at a corporate training site. Many reps do not even understand basic medical terminology, much less how to convince a doctor to prescribe a drug. They might not even know anything about the company. Corporate training serves as a kind of initiation ritual. "They have to professionalize you in some way," says Oldani. "You can't go in cold turkey or you'd be a bumbling idiot." The first phase of training for Oldani was in Chicago, but it was a later session near Princeton, New Jersey, that he remembers as the most effective. "That was three weeks where you go to a corporate training facility, complete isolation, and there is a real attempt to totally indoctrinate you into what you're going to be doing," he says. Picture a cohort of young, attractive men and women, plucked out of small towns in Wisconsin or North Carolina, and transported to an expensive hotel near Princeton, where they will spend every day for three weeks in the company of one another—learning the ins and outs of detailing a doctor, taking part in hokey bonding exercises, and finishing off the day with happy hour. Competition was heartily encouraged. Reps paired off to play volleyball and softball for prizes. They worked on their presentations in teams. They were shown the awards they could win if they did their jobs well. Oldani makes it sound like a blend of sales convention, boot camp, and college spring break. "And then you are slowly introduced to the award winners," Oldani says. "That's the key thing about training. Reps would come in from around the country, and it would be: 'This is five-time VPC winner from Macon County, Georgia—Sam Bellafonte!' And then he'd get up there and give his spiel, and he'd work with you on the side. You'd watch videos of these reps, and then: they're there! The superstars, the all-star sellers."

After each corporate-site training session the rookie rep returned to his or her home territory for practical field experience with a regional manager. "My first manager was like *Glengarry Glen Ross,* but on a funny, more absurdist scale," says Oldani. "He was old school." Pacing around the room, the manager would point to one rep after another, comparing their performances. "He'd talk bonus," Oldani says. "A lot of managers wouldn't share what other reps made. But he'd be like 'Max, why don't you tell the group what you won?' And Max stands up and says, 'Well, I got these coupons, and I'm going to get a set of golf clubs, some new shoes'—and he cuts him off and says, 'Yeah, that's great. Mikey, tell him what you won.' And I say, 'I won ten grand.'" The message was clear: if you're really doing your job, you're collecting extra cash.

When Oldani talks about his early days with Pfizer he portrays himself as a young rube from the Midwest, star-struck by the big-time pharma company, awed by the mere prospect of a free car. "I can remember being real Squaresville. I didn't own good suits, and I came walking in one time with a cloth tie on." He starts grinning. "You know, these were hard-core dudes. They were cool and liked me, but still, it was: 'Nice cloth tie, Oldani! Where are you from, Gomer?' I didn't know anything about Johnston and Murphy shoes, or cuffed and pleated pants. You can believe when I went back I got the right outfits." The new job created some tension back home too. "I remember my dad making comments to me too, like 'Ah, Mr. Big-Time Salesman,'" Oldani says. "He was the one who encouraged me to get the job, and he was already kind of ribbing me, because the salesmen he dealt with he never really liked. He thought they were phony. He says, 'So are you going to start wearing pinkie rings?' And I remember thinking: *My God, there* are *a lot of guys with pinkie rings.* Class rings were big, army rings, award rings. You could get a ring if you won Vice President's Club, kind of like a Super Bowl ring."

Oldani developed his own approach, one that turned less on the hard sell than on personal relationships. He brings up a phrase coined by the French theorist Pierre Bourdieu during his fieldwork in Algeria: "the man of good faith."[21] When economic transactions take place among strangers, all of whom know little about the motives, character, or tactics of one another, it is very easy to be tricked or cheated. But one way to overcome that lack of knowledge is trust. If you can trust the person you are doing business with—if, say, he is vouched for by someone you know well—he is a "man of good faith." Doing business with a man of good faith is a little like doing business with a friend or relative. You have confidence that he will not take advantage of you because your relationship is social and personal rather than purely economic. "Walking in a clinic back door," says Oldani. "That's a man of good faith." Over time some doctors came to trust Oldani so much that they got into the habit of calling him about new drugs or their side effects. "To me, that was total faith, good confidence," Oldani says. "They didn't want a clinical trial; they didn't want me to bring the data in; they just wanted to talk to me on the phone." An especially impressive example took place not long ago as Oldani was making plans to go out for the evening with a psychiatrist friend. "Their babysitter was the Lilly rep!" Oldani says, scarcely hiding his astonishment. "I thought: *Wow, now that's total confidence.* 'I trust my child to this drug rep.'"

Oldani has spent so much time thinking about gifts partly because of the role they'd played in helping him establish social relationships. "Social exchanges are humanizing, pure economic exchanges dehumanizing," explains Oldani. His goal was to move from the economic realm to the social, which may be why he was uncomfortable with the formal, routinized sales tactics. Oldani never used much script-tracking data, and he could not bring himself to close his detailing visits with "Can I count on you to write prescriptions for Zoloft for your next five patients?" Over time, though, the drug business began to move toward a more purely economic model: closely audited, impersonal, driven by numbers, specifically targeted at high prescribers. Eventually, when Oldani walked into an office, it wasn't "Hey, it's Mike." It was "Hey, it's another Pfizer rep."

Oldani used to call on a hospital pharmacist who really knew how to work the system. "That guy was a closer," Oldani says. "He knew how to get reps in his office and put the pressure on you. All of a sudden you're buying a thousand dollars' of raffle tickets, or three coolers and chicken for a picnic." For years the pharmacist had been called on by a Pfizer rep called Gary, a bland figure who had eventually left to become a manager. He was replaced by a second Pfizer rep whom the pharmacist called "Gary Two." He did the same things the first Gary did, but upped it a notch or two. When Oldani eventually replaced that rep, he became "Gary Three." Oldani says, "To be a Gary in that hospital meant, if you did so many favors for him, he let you walk around the hospital, which was supposed to be closed. I'd go up to the ICU. I'd go up to surgery." He pauses for minute and says, "I think I was his best Gary."

• • •

A few years ago a small group of first-year medical students at the University of Minnesota spoke to me about a lecture on erectile dysfunction that had just been given by a member of the urology department. The doctor's PowerPoint slides had a large, watermarked logo in the corner. At one point during the lecture a student raised his hand and, somewhat disingenuously, asked the urologist to explain the logo. The urologist, caught off guard, stumbled for a moment and then said that it was the logo for Cialis, a drug for erectile dysfunction that is manufactured by Eli Lilly. Another student asked if he had a special relationship with Eli Lilly. The urologist replied that yes, he was on the advisory board for the company, which had supplied the slides. But he quickly added that nobody needed to worry about the objectivity of his lecture, because he was also on the advisory boards of the makers of the competing drugs Viagra and Levitra. The second student told me, "A lot of people agreed that it was a pharm lecture and that we should have gotten a free breakfast."

This episode is not as unusual as it might appear. Drug company–sponsored consultancies, advisory-board memberships, and speaking engagements have become so common, especially among medical-school faculty, that the urologist probably never imagined that he would be challenged for lecturing to medical students with materials produced by Eli Lilly. According to a recent study in the *Journal of the American Medical Association,* nine out of ten medical students have been asked or required by an attending physician to go to a lunch sponsored by a drug company.[22]

Over the past several years pharmaceutical profits have started to level off, and a backlash against reps has been felt; some companies have reduced their sales forces. But the industry as a whole has been hiring more and more doctors as speakers. In 2004, it sponsored nearly twice as many educational events led by doctors as ones led by reps. Not long before, the numbers had been roughly equal. This raises a question: Are doctors becoming the new drug reps?

Doctors are often the best people to market a drug to other doctors. Merck discovered this when it was developing a campaign for Vioxx, before the drug was taken off the market because of its association with heart attacks and strokes. According to an internal study by Merck, reported in the *Wall Street Journal*, doctors who attended a lecture given by another doctor subsequently wrote nearly four times more prescriptions for Vioxx than doctors who attended an event led by a rep. The return on investment for doctor-led events was nearly twice that of rep-led events, even after subtracting the generous fees Merck paid to the doctors who spoke.[23]

These speaking invitations work much like gifts. While reps hope, of course, that a doctor who is speaking on behalf of their company will give their drugs good PR, they also know that this doctor is more likely to write prescriptions for their drugs. "If he didn't write, he wouldn't speak," a rep who has worked for four pharmaceutical companies told me. The semi-official industry term for these speakers and consultants is *thought leaders*, or *key opinion leaders*. Some thought leaders do not stay loyal to one company but generate a tidy supplemental income by speaking and consulting for a number of different companies. Reps refer to these doctors as "drug whores."

The seduction, whether by one company or several, is often quite gradual. My brother Hal explained to me how he wound up on the speakers' bureau of a major pharmaceutical company. It started when a company rep asked him if he'd be interested in giving a talk about clinical depression to a community group. The honorarium was a thousand dollars. Hal thought, *Why not?* It seemed almost a public service. The next time, the company asked him to talk not to the public but to practitioners at a community hospital. Soon company reps were making suggestions about content. "Why don't you mention the side-effect profiles of the different antidepressants?" they asked. Uneasy, Hal tried to ignore these suggestions. Still, the more talks he gave, the more the reps became focused on antidepressants rather than depression. The company began giving him PowerPoint slides to use, which he also ignored. The reps started telling him, "You know, we have you on the local circuit giving these talks, but you're medical-school faculty; we could get you on the national circuit. That's where the real money is." The mention of big money made him even more uneasy. Eventually the reps asked him to lecture about a new version of their antidepressant drug. Soon after that, Hal told them, "I can't do this anymore."

Looking back on this trajectory, Hal said, "It's kind of like you're a woman at a party, and your boss says to you, 'Look, do me a favor: be nice to this guy over there.' And you see the guy is not bad-looking, and you're unattached, so you say, 'Why not? I can be nice.'" The problem is that it never ends with that party. "Soon you find yourself on the way to a Bangkok brothel in the cargo hold of an unmarked plane. And you say, 'Whoa, this is not what I agreed to.' But then you have to ask yourself, 'When did the prostitution actually start? Wasn't it at that party?'"

Some believe that the marketing landscape changed dramatically for both reps and doctors in 2002, after the Office of Inspector General in the Department of Health and Human Services announced its intention to crack down on drug companies' more notorious promotional practices. With the threat of prosecution in the air, the industry began to take the job of self-policing a lot more seriously, and PhRMA issued a set of voluntary marketing guidelines. Those guidelines specified, for example, that spouses of doctors should not be given free meals, and that gifts should be worth less than a hundred dollars and be for the benefit of patients. PhRMA updated the voluntary code again in 2009.

Although most reps agree that the PhRMA code has changed things, not all of them agree that it changed things for the better. Some say that as long as reps feel pressure to meet quota, they will find ways to get around the rules. As one former rep pointed out, not all drug companies belong to PhRMA, and those that don't are, of course, not bound by PhRMA's guidelines. Jordan Katz says that things actually got worse after 2002. "The companies that tried to follow the guidelines lost a ton of market share, and the ones who didn't gained it," he says. "The bottom line is that if you don't pay off the doctors, you will not succeed in pharmaceuticals. Period."

• • •

In 1997, John Lantos, a pediatrician and ethicist at the University of Chicago, wrote a book called *Do We Still Need Doctors?*[24] We will always need health care, of course. But, as Lantos observes, it is not clear that we will always need to get our health care from doctors. Many of us already get it from other providers—nurses, physical therapists, clinical psychologists, nutritionists, respiratory therapists, and so on. The figure of "the doctor" is not cast in stone. It is really just a particular configuration of roles and duties and responsibilities, each of which can be changed.

Many have already been changed. Sometimes I think of my father as one of the last small-town, solo family doctors left in America. His kind of practice has been largely replaced by teams of specialists working in group practices underwritten by insurance companies and for-profit health-care chains. I doubt that any of the doctors my family has ever visited, except for a pediatrician who took care of our children when we lived in Montreal, would recognize us if he or she passed us in the street. A few years ago, while driving in Wisconsin, I filled up my car at a combination gas station, pharmacy, and walk-in medical clinic. I don't mean to complain. As long as the health insurance is paid up, my family and I usually get good care. We simply live in a country that has decided that the traditional figure of the doctor is not worth preserving in the face of modern economics. Instead, we Americans put our trust in the market.

Perhaps we are right to do so. People can get used to a world without doctors. As Lantos points out, we have gotten used to a world where we have shoes but no cobblers. We can copy documents without scriveners, make tools without blacksmiths, and produce books in the absence of bookbinders. We have left the old world behind, and for the most part, we don't miss it.

As the figure of the traditional doctor fades away, it is being replaced by a figure akin to the drug rep, one whose responsibility is to compete as vigorously as possible in the medical marketplace. Patients are being replaced by health-care consumers, who shop for the best medical bargains they can find. If it is true that the drug rep does not put an individual patient's interests first, the same is true of everyone else selling in the marketplace; and we believe that such problems in the marketplace will be sorted out by the invisible hand. Buyers will stop buying from sellers who provide them with inferior goods. This model of medicine is not unlike that advocated thirty years ago by Robert Sade, a surgeon at my old medical school, the Medical University of South Carolina. Writing in the *New England Journal of Medicine,* Sade argued, "Medical care is neither a right nor a privilege: it is a service provided by doctors and others to people who wish to purchase it."[25] Sade later became chair of the AMA's Council of Ethical and Judicial Affairs.

Many doctors seem resigned to this shift. They see themselves as members of a beleaguered group whose lives are made miserable by third-party payers, personal-injury attorneys, and hospital bureaucrats. Whatever idealism they may have had about the practice of medicine is being pushed aside by the concrete realities of hustling in the new medical marketplace. Many academic physicians seem cowed by the power of the drug companies, upon whom a number depend for research funding. For some, it's not so much a question of whether medicine has become a business as what kind of business it has become. When I talked recently to a gastroenterologist at an Ivy League medical school about his work as a thought leader for a variety of drug companies, he shrugged and said, "Better a whore than a concubine."

Which is not to say that pockets of resistance can't be found, especially among younger physicians and medical students. The American Medical Student Association is one of the few mainstream medical organizations with a principled position against taking industry gifts. It stands in striking contrast to the American Academy of Family Physicians, which recently refused to grant exhibition space at its annual conference to No Free Lunch, a physician-led advocacy group that advises physicians to "Just say no to drug reps." The AAFP said that the group's goals were "not within the character and purpose" of the conference. But it allowed pharmaceutical companies, McDonald's, and the Distilled Spirits Council of the United States to exhibit. (It reversed its decision about No Free Lunch after protests by a number of AAFP members.)[26]

Whether doctors and reps are all that different from each other is no longer clear. Doctors know a lot more about medicine, and drug reps dress a lot better, but these days both are Organization Men, small cogs in a vast health-care machine. They are just doing their jobs in a market-driven health-care bureaucracy that Americans have designed and that we defend vigorously to critics elsewhere in the world. Like anyone else, doctors and reps are responding to the pressures and incentives of the system in which they work.

When Michael Oldani and I were having breakfast, he told me a story about a rep he'd interviewed for his dissertation. The rep had recently spent a day doing a preceptorship, a practice in which a drug company pays doctors to let reps shadow them while they see patients. This rep was shadowing a high-prescribing psychiatrist (she called him Dr. C) at a med-check clinic. Med-check clinics are extremely busy sites where psychiatrists see large numbers of patients in quick succession, mainly to make sure that their medications are in proper order. At one point during the day, the rep said, a cheerful man in a wheelchair rolled into the office. Barely looking up from the stack of charts on his desk, Dr. C started quizzing the man about his medications. After a few minutes the man interrupted. "Look at me, Dr. C. Notice anything different?" Dr. C pushed his glasses up on top of his head and looked carefully at the patient for a few seconds before replying, "No, I don't. What's up?" The man smiled and said excitedly, "I got my legs cut off!"

After a moment of silence, Dr. C smiled. The man laughed. Neither seemed upset. In a few minutes the session ended, and the next patient came in.

CHAPTER FOUR

The Thought Leaders

I N THE EARLY 1970S, a group of medical researchers decided to
study an unusual question: How would a medical audience respond to a lecture that was completely devoid of content yet delivered with authority by a convincing phony? To find out, the authors hired
a distinguished-looking actor and gave him the name Dr. Myron L. Fox.
They fabricated an impressive CV for Dr. Fox and billed him as an expert
in mathematics and human behavior. Finally, they provided him with
a fake lecture composed largely of impressive-sounding gibberish and
titled "Mathematical Game Theory as Applied to Physician Education"
and had him wear a white coat and deliver the lecture to three separate
medical audiences. At the end of each lecture, the audience members
filled out a survey questionnaire.

The responses were overwhelmingly positive. The audience members described Dr. Fox with adjectives such as *extremely articulate* and
captivating. Another said he delivered "a very dramatic presentation."
After one lecture, 90 percent of the audience members said they'd found
the talk by Dr. Fox "stimulating." Overall, almost every member of every audience loved Dr. Fox's lecture, despite the fact that, as the authors
write, it was delivered by an actor "programmed to teach charismatically
and non-substantively on a topic about which he knew nothing."[1]

It is tempting to imagine that the Dr. Fox study reveals a deep flaw
in the structure of medicine—that health-care workers are too trust-
ing of authority, for example, or that Continuing Medical Education is
somehow a sham. But what the stories actually reveal may be something
closer to the opposite. If medicine were simple and transparent, pretending to be a medical expert would be very difficult. An audience could

spot incompetence right away. Pretending to be a medical expert is possible precisely because medical knowledge is so specialized and opaque. These days an ordinary doctor can no more expect to understand the intricacies of specialized medical research than the driveway mechanic who tinkered with his Volkswagen in 1962 can expect to fully understand the complex, computerized automobiles on the road today. Anyone who has tried to sit through a medical lecture in a field other than his own will secretly admit that he probably would have been fooled by Dr. Fox as well.

Since the 1950s, marketers have been taken with the idea that when it comes to spreading the word about unfamiliar products or concepts, some people are far more important than others. The term *opinion leader* was made familiar by the sociologists Paul Lazarsfeld and Elihu Katz in their 1955 book *Personal Influence*, where they used the term to explain the way that media messages were filtered and spread by personal, face-to-face contact with influential people.[2] It is not hard to see why marketers liked this idea. Mass-media advertising can be expensive. What if there was a way to avoid the masses and simply concentrate on the special people? Today the pharmaceutical industry uses the terms *key opinion leader* (KOL) and *thought leader* to refer to influential physicians, often academic researchers, who are especially effective at transmitting messages to their peers. Pharmaceutical companies hire KOLs to consult for them, to give lectures, and, occasionally, to make presentations on their behalf at regulatory meetings or hearings.

The KOL is a combination of celebrity spokesperson, neighborhood gossip, and the popular kid in high school. KOLs do not exactly endorse drugs, at least not in ways that are too obvious, but their opinions can be used to market them—sometimes by word of mouth, but more often by quasi-academic activities, such as grand-rounds lectures, sponsored symposia, and articles in medical journals. While pharmaceutical companies seek out high-status KOLs with impressive academic appointments, status is only one determinant of a KOL's influence. Just as important is the fact that a KOL is, at least in theory, independent. Medical audiences trusted Dr. Fox partly because he played the role of an expert so convincingly: white coat, gray hair, and a complicated lecture delivered with authority. But they also trusted him because they had no reason *not* to trust him. Dr. Fox was not selling a product or pitching an idea. The very implausibility of his charade is part of what made it so persuasive. Dr. Fox appeared to be impartial.

It is not hard to see why pharmaceutical companies would like to have a Dr. Fox speaking on their behalf. Most marketers would like to have a convincing, influential, and apparently independent expert who will deliver the text given to him. The more interesting question is: Why do so many academic physicians want to be Dr. Fox?

• • •

"It strokes your narcissism," says Dr. Erick Turner, a psychiatrist at the University of Oregon. There is the money, of course, which is no small matter. Some high-level KOLs make more money consulting for industry than they get from their academic institutions. But the real appeal of being a KOL is that of being acknowledged as important. That feeling of importance comes not so much from the pharmaceutical companies themselves but from associating with other academic luminaries that the companies have recruited. Academic physicians talk about the experience of being a KOL the way others might talk about being admitted to a selective fraternity or an exclusive New York dance club. No longer are you standing outside the rope line trying to catch the doorman's eye, waiting hungrily to be admitted. You are one of the chosen. "You get to hobnob with these mega thought leaders and these aspiring thought leaders," Turner says. "They make you feel like you're special."

Turner is a former drug reviewer for the FDA. He worked at the FDA for three years, after six years as a fellow at the National Institute of Mental Health. In 2003, after taking an academic position at Oregon, he began giving talks on behalf of pharmaceutical companies—Eli Lilly, AstraZeneca, and Bristol-Myers Squibb. "I left the FDA, and I felt kind of frustrated that I had all this knowledge about how clinical trials work, and I felt there wasn't much of anything I could do with it," says Turner. "It felt like a demotion going from bossing big pharma around, where you tell them to jump and they ask how high, and then suddenly you are way on the other end of the food chain. You're begging to be a site investigator, and they say, 'Nah, I don't think so. You might have trouble recruiting,' or 'Your IRB is too slow.'"

Actually doing clinical trials for drug companies is often boring, Turner says. The companies design the trial protocols and hire investigators to conduct them at many different locations. A given clinical investigator has no real influence. But if you are involved with the rollout of a new drug, you are really in on the action. "The first thing they do is ferry you to a really nice hotel," says Turner. "And sometimes they pick you up in a limo, and you feel very important, and they have really, really good food. And they make you sign a confidentiality agreement and say you need to sign this if you want to get paid." The meetings Turner attended featured what he calls "mega thought leaders," the recognized leaders in the field, who gave presentations to a group of people like him—the second-tier "little thought leaders." ("It was kind of like the farm team," he says.) The companies will also offer these aspiring thought leaders media training and advice on public speaking. "They give you slides that you will probably be speaking from, and you'll be in a room with about a dozen other people," Turner says. "You get up there, and you have your pointer, and then you stand off to the side when you're done. And the facilitator will say, 'So what did you think of his voice? What did you think of his body language? Did he project well?'"

It is an article of faith among pharmaceutical executives that KOLs are a critical part of any marketing plan. According to a 2004 study of the fifteen largest pharmaceutical companies, the industry spends just under a third of total marketing expenditures on KOLs.[3] So important are KOLs that new businesses have emerged solely to recruit, train, and manage them, such as Skila, OpenQ, and pharMethod. The influence of KOLs is thought to be strongest when a new drug is being launched, but the industry also steps up spending when other changes occur, such as the launch of a competitor drug or new evidence about a damaging side effect.

The reason KOLs are so important is their role in managing the discourse around a given product—a discourse that is equal parts scientific study, commercial hype, and academic buzz. That discourse will begin years before a drug or device is launched, and it will usually continue at least until the patent expires. Television and magazine ads aside, the primary locus of this discourse is scientific communication—journal articles, medical conferences, grand-rounds lectures, lunch and dinner meetings, and CME events. Virtually all physicians are on the receiving end of communication, but only a relatively few deliver it. If the industry can influence those few, then it can also influence the rest.

Thought leaders serve an indispensable function when it comes to a potentially very lucrative marketing niche: off-label promotion. Doctors are given wide latitude to prescribe drugs for any condition the drug might help, but pharmaceutical companies can promote the drugs only for the conditions for which the FDA has approved them. So while an AstraZeneca rep can talk to a doctor about, say, the antipsychotic drug Seroquel (quetiapine) for schizophrenia, a condition the FDA has approved Seroquel to treat, the rep would be strictly forbidden to suggest that a doctor might try the drug for patients with insomnia. Yet off-label marketing is tempting; some drugs generate far more revenue from off-label prescriptions than they do for their approved indications. One recent study found that over 80 percent of prescriptions for the anti-seizure drug Neurontin (gabapentin) and the antidepressant Elavil (amitriptyline) were for off-label uses. The same study showed that for most off-label uses, there was little or no scientific support.[4]

Off-label promotion is a topic that makes many industry employees visibly nervous. It is a very effective piece of prescription-generating machinery, and rumor has it that many managers encourage it—but if a drug rep is caught promoting a drug off-label, he or she could be fired. Off-label marketing can also be costly. For example, Lilly recently settled a $1.4 billion suit for off-label marketing of Zyprexa (olanzapine), an anti-psychotic drug approved to treat schizophrenia and bipolar disorder but which Lilly was allegedly promoting as a tool for calming agitated elderly patients with dementia.[5]

Companies use a range of familiar tricks to get around the ban on off-label promotion, many of them aimed at generating buzz about the product.[6] The case of Neurontin is instructive. In 1996 a whistle-blower named David Franklin, a medical-science liaison with Parke-Davis (now a division of Pfizer), filed suit against the company over its off-label pro-motion of this drug. Neurontin was approved as an adjunct treatment of epilepsy, but according to the lawsuit, Parke-Davis was promoting it for other conditions—including bipolar disorder, migraines, and restless legs syndrome—for which there was little or no scientific evidence that the drug worked. "We all know Neurontin's not growing adjunctive ther-apy," said a Parke-Davis marketing executive caught on tape. "Besides, that is not where the money is. Pain management, now that's money." The executive told his medical-science liaisons, "That's where we need to be holding their hand and whispering in their ear, Neurontin for pain, Neurontin for monotherapy, Neurontin for bipolar, Neurontin for every-thing."[7]

To market Neurontin off-label, the company employed a variety of schemes, most involving a combination of rep ingenuity and payments to KOLs. Some KOLs signed ghostwritten journal articles. One received more than $300,000 to speak about Neurontin at conferences. Others were paid just to listen. (Simply having some of your KOLs in attendance at a dinner meeting is valuable, explains Kathleen Slattery-Moschkau, a former drug rep, because thought leaders will often bring up off-label uses of a drug without having to be prompted. "You can't get a better selling situation than that," she says.) The litigation over Neurontin cost

Pfizer $430 million in criminal fines and civil damages for the period of 1994 to 2002. But the cost was well worth it. The drug's popularity and profitability soared. In spite of the adverse publicity, Neurontin generated more than $2.7 billion in revenues in 2003, 90 percent of which came from off-label prescriptions.[8]

Turner began giving talks to community doctors, often in the evenings over dinner. A step up from dinner meetings were officially sanctioned CME events, such as grand-rounds presentations. Up another notch were the lectures to psychiatrists and other specialists at professional conferences, often at satellite symposia—industry-funded sessions that ran alongside the peer-reviewed presentations. Pharmaceutical companies frequently collect the papers from these sessions and publish them in supplements to medical journals. Turner gave industry talks for about a year and a half before giving it up. "It starts to dawn on you. You think: is this what I thought it would be? It's like signing up for a job or a marriage that doesn't work out. It takes you a while to admit that this isn't what you were hoping for."

Turner says he became frustrated with the limitations placed on what he could say. By the time he began speaking, in the mid-2000s, the companies had begun to worry about being nailed for off-label marketing. "In the old days they used to be a lot more free and easy about what speakers could do, but they've gotten tighter and tighter, for fear of getting their hands slapped by the FDA." Turner was given slides prepared by the company and was warned not to deviate from the slides. "They would really drum that into us—oh, this slide set has been vetted by the FDA, and we've got to be very careful. We can't say anything that's not in the slide set—*unless* someone asks a question that is unsolicited. And then you can bring in your own clinical experience, and give your own interpretation. But you can't volunteer it up front." Turner says the experience was similar to the problem he had doing industry-funded clinical trials. "They have a protocol figured out, it's all done, they have it cleared with the FDA, and they say: 'Do you want to do it or not?' And with the speaking, it is: 'Here's the talk: do you want to give it or not?'"

Turner's observation appears to be a fairly common one. Litigation and bad publicity have pressed the pharmaceutical industry into retreating from many marketing practices that became commonplace during the 1990s, especially those involving paid speakers. Daniel Metzger (a pseudonym) is a gastroenterologist at an elite medical school who has been giving talks for the pharmaceutical industry for decades. "In the old days, I would only do a visiting-speaker talk if they let me bring my own slides," he says. "I used to say, 'I am not prepared to use your crappy slides which are just pure regurgitations of your own studies, which are not that interesting anyway, and which make me look like a spokesperson for the company.'" Back then the pharmaceutical companies would concede to Metzger's wishes, allowing him to speak on his own terms. These days, however, the companies are much more cautious. "The pharma companies are terrified that somebody might say the wrong thing in a room and a mole will pick it up and they will get blackballed by the FDA." Metzger still gives industry-funded CME talks, which he believes are legitimate, but he no longer gives talks as a member of a speakers' bureau. He says, "This is essentially FDA-approved marketing, except that it comes out of a doctor's mouth."

The status of being a KOL carries a certain irony. It is a hunger for status that motivates many academic physicians to work for industry, yet in order to preserve their status, those physicians must also cultivate the perception of their independence. Nobody respects an academic who does not think for himself. If Dr. Fox had been unmasked as an actor merely reading his lines, nobody would have paid any attention. And of course, most academics do not especially want to think of themselves as figures like Dr. Fox, merely reciting lines that have been written by someone else. As Turner asks, "Is it worth it, feeling like you are a robot, just speaking from a pre-fab slide set?"

Given the intense public scrutiny of high-profile thought leaders in recent years, it would be easy to conclude that the phenomenon of cultivating thought leaders is new. Yet nothing could be further from the truth. Pharmaceutical companies have been using thought leaders to market their products for at least fifty years. In fact, one of the most controversial pharmaceutical marketing bonanzas of the past half century owes its genesis largely to a single, highly influential man.

•   •   •

In 1966, Robert Wilson, a Brooklyn gynecologist, published a book called *Feminine Forever*.[9] Mainly a collection of personal stories from Wilson's practice, *Feminine Forever* reported the remarkable antiaging effects of estrogen replacement therapy. Wilson had given estrogen to more than five thousand women to protect them from withering away at menopause, a period of life that, as he put it, turns a woman into a "dull-minded but sharp-tongued caricature of her former self." Estrogen, he predicted, would keep a woman vibrant and desirable into her later years. *Feminine Forever* sold a hundred thousand copies in six months. Within a year, it was available in seventeen countries.

The manufacturers of estrogen replacement therapy were fully aware of how valuable a commodity Wilson was, as Sheila and David Rothman note in their perceptive history of medical enhancement *The Pursuit of Perfection*.[10] Two years earlier, the makers of Premarin, Enovid, and Provera had given Wilson a $31,350 "research grant" to establish an antiaging foundation. Never in his life had Wilson held an academic post, but between April 1963 and August 1964 he published thirteen articles in medical journals arguing the benefits of estrogen. His Wilson Research Foundation arranged lectures and distributed pamphlets promoting estrogen therapy and even kept a list of doctors who prescribed estrogen. Wilson became a recognizable figure in the popular media, telling women in magazines like *Look* and *Vogue* how estrogen would make them "grow visibly younger day by day."

Many women began asking their gynecologists for estrogen. "They've all read Dr. Wilson's book and all the magazine articles about estrogen, and they insist that I give them the pills," said one Miami gynecologist. Given the effects of estrogen that women were reporting, this was no surprise. "After two and a half weeks, I awoke one morning with a sense of well-being I'd never experienced before," said one. Another said, "It is a miracle to find myself at the age of 71 enjoying better health after several years of misery. I am stronger, my vision has improved, and I have experienced an orgasm."

Men were happy too. In fact, the pharmaceutical industry often advertised estrogen to doctors in a way that emphasized its benefits for men. "Menrium treats the menopausal symptoms that bother him the most" declared the advertisements from Roche. Ayerst ran ads with the tagline "He is suffering from menopause because of her." Because menopause was thought to be associated with depression and anxiety, some pharmaceutical companies bundled estrogen and a "minor tranquilizer" into a single pill. Wallace Laboratories marketed Milprem, a combination of estrogen and Miltown, while Roche produced a combination of estrogen and Librium.

Central to the marketing of estrogen in the 1960s was what Alastair Matheson calls a "drug narrative"—a story weaving together the central marketing threads a company wants to communicate about a product, which are then reinforced by the company's thought leaders.[11] Initially these drug narratives presented estrogen not as a medical treatment but as a natural replacement for what a woman's body began failing to produce at menopause. Wilson emphasized this point in his lectures and publications. "Estrogen therapy doesn't *change* a woman," wrote Wilson. "*[I]t keeps her from changing*, that is, from suffering 'living decay.' " The enthusiasm of clinicians for estrogen therapy was matched by a body of research data that, while more cautious than articles in the popular press, appeared to demonstrate that estrogen had a clear medical benefit.

Estrogen manufacturers were forced to change the narrative after 1974, when a study in the *New England Journal of Medicine* suggested that estrogen might be linked to a heightened risk of endometrial cancer. This study was followed by a warning from the Food and Drug Administration, and the number of prescriptions for estrogen replacement therapy dropped from twenty-seven million in 1975 to fourteen million in 1980. Yet over the next twenty years or so, the use of estrogens gradually crept back up. Manufacturers began combining estrogen with progesterone, and the name was changed from "estrogen replacement therapy" to "hormone replacement therapy." The narrative shifted away from hormones as a natural replacement aimed at postponing aging and toward the idea that hormones were a type of preventive medicine. This narrative was based on data suggesting that hormones helped prevent cardiovascular disease and osteoporosis. In time, this narrative would prove very successful. By the 1990s, it was estimated that about a third of postmenopausal women were taking hormone replacement therapy.

In July 2002 there came a dramatic reversal. The largest clinical trial of hormone replacement therapy ever conducted was stopped prematurely because hormones were proving to be so risky. In 1993 the National Institutes of Health had started the Women's Health Initiative (WHI), one piece of which was a large study of hormone replacement therapy. The plan was to recruit sixty-five thousand women to take hormone therapies and compare these women with a hundred thousand controls. The trial was supposed to run until 2005, but when the safety and monitoring board analyzed the data in 2002, it found that health outcomes were so poor for women on hormone replacement therapy that the board could not in good conscience allow women in the study to keep taking it.[12] As the Rothmans summarize the trial: "Over one year, 10,000 women taking estrogen plus progestin compared to placebo would experience 7 more coronary artery disease events, 8 more strokes, 8 more pulmonary blood clots, and 8 more invasive breast cancers . . ." The study stunned many doctors and was widely reported in the popular press, including cover stories in *Time* and *Newsweek*. So thoroughly had most physicians been convinced of the drug narrative that it never occurred to them that it might not be true.

In some ways, Wilson was an unusual thought leader for the hormone replacement campaign. He was not an academic physician, and until he was chosen by the estrogen manufacturers, he had not published any medical research. Yet he became a medical celebrity. Wilson's rise to prominence suggests an important lesson. The industry does not merely recruit thought leaders; it has the ability to create them. Today that ability is even greater than it was in Wilson's era. Pharmaceutical companies can fund the research of aspiring thought leaders, put them on scientific programs, make them investigators on clinical trials, make arrangements for them to give CME events, fund their travel, and manage their "authorship" of journal articles. "They will figure out how to polish you as an opinion leader," says Peter Whitehouse, a neurologist at Case Western Reserve University who worked for many years as a thought leader before cutting his industry ties. "I got to do lots of things because they were grooming me."

There was a time in the past when the locus of status in medicine resided in its elite academic institutions, like the Mayo Clinic and the Johns Hopkins Medical School. Pharmaceutical companies wanted desperately to attach themselves to these institutions in the hope of sharing a little of their prestige. Today, however, status in the medical world is much more complicated. It is not that status has moved from academic medicine to pharmaceutical companies. (In fact, the reputation of the pharmaceutical industry among the general public has rarely been lower.) But pharmaceutical companies hold the money and political power. And because pharmaceutical companies are so widely distrusted by the public, they need academic physicians to front their research and give it a patina of legitimacy. What academic physicians need is industry money, especially at a time when struggling academic health centers are pressing their faculty members to become "revenue generators." Academics are like fading European aristocrats who are so strapped for cash that they have turned their stately homes into museums for gum-chewing American tourists and must contemplate selling their titles.

The academic physicians' values have also changed. "There used to be disdain among academics toward the commercial sector," says Bob Whitaker, a journalist and cofounder of CenterWatch. Until the 1990s, academic physicians actually helped design trials for the industry; they didn't just put their names on articles and front presentations. Industry had to approach academics with hat in hand to get them to be involved. But as trials moved to the commercial sector, universities began behaving more like businesses in order to compete. Whitaker says, "Academics realized that in this new commercial environment, their credentials were marketable."

The pharmaceutical industry has proved to be a willing buyer. Yet given the amount of time and money the industry invests in thought leaders—identifying them, recruiting them, buffing and polishing them—it is worth asking: Where does all this confidence in the power of thought leaders originate? There are many different ways to spend a marketing budget. Where did the pharmaceutical industry get the idea that this one was so important?

• • •

In the mid-1950s, three sociologists with a research grant from Pfizer set out for the Midwest in search of an answer to a simple question: What makes a doctor decide to start using a new drug—or, as they put it more generally, a "medical innovation"? How does the use of that medical innovation spread through the medical community? One of the sociologists, Elihu Katz, had helped develop the two-step-flow model of communication with his Columbia University mentor Paul Lazarsfeld. In their book *Personal Influence*, they contested the popular notion that people simply absorb messages directly from the mass media like beachgoers absorb sunshine. Instead, media messages are filtered through people who pass the messages on to others. Particularly important are the charmed individuals who, by virtue of their authority, charisma, or social relationships, have a special gift for message transmission. Katz and Lazarsfeld called these people "influentials."

Personal Influence concerned messages about things like movies and fashion. Were messages about new medical therapies transmitted in the same way? In *Medical Innovation*, Katz and his colleagues James Coleman and Herbert Menzel tracked messages about a particular new drug, tetracycline.[13] Tetracycline is an antibiotic that is widely used today, but fifty years ago it was just being introduced to the market. The area they studied consisted of four midwestern communities. The largest was a city of 110,000 people with 182 doctors and three hospitals, two of them teaching hospitals. The other communities were located nearby but were smaller, with populations of 30,000 to 40,000 people and between 45 and 75 doctors. The sociologists used local pharmacy and hospital records to track prescriptions for tetracycline.

Because the sociologists were interested especially in the effects of social networks, they did not merely do general interviews with doctors. They asked the doctors three specific questions. First: To whom do you turn when you need advice? Second: With whom do you discuss cases or treatments? And third: With which doctors do you socialize? The answers they received varied dramatically. Some doctors were located squarely in the center of medical life. They shared offices with other doctors, had regular hospital appointments, went to lots of professional meetings, and had lots of friends in the medical community. But other doctors were relatively isolated. They practiced solo, had only courtesy privileges at the hospitals, and kept to themselves socially, at least in relation to other doctors. The sociologists used these measures of social connectedness to create a series of maps with which they tracked the spread of tetracycline use.

In the early period after tetracycline came onto the market, the sociologists found little difference in tetracycline prescriptions between the socially integrated doctors and the isolated doctors. Soon, however, the number of socially integrated doctors prescribing tetracycline began to accelerate. The more contacts a socially integrated doctor had, the more opportunities that doctor had to spread the word about tetracycline. In contrast, among the isolated doctors, who had far fewer opportunities to transmit the message, the rate of tetracycline adoption stayed relatively flat. To the sociologists, this pattern of transmission resembled the outbreak of an infectious disease. Receiving a message was less like getting a tan than it was like getting the flu. Each person got the infection from someone else.

The sociologists distinguished between two stages in the communication of new information. In the awareness stage, doctors are simply informed about a new drug. This kind of information can be transmitted by direct mail or detailing. But in the evaluation stage, communication actually *legitimates* the use of the drug. It is in the evaluation stage that peer-to-peer interactions become far more important than information. In situations of uncertainty where the correct course of action is unclear, people generally turn to others for guidance. The sociologists in *Medical Innovation* called this "social contagion," but in fact it may be closer to social conformity. The more embedded in the medical community doctors were, the greater the social pressure they felt to prescribe tetracycline.

Either way, the effects of social networks appeared early. They were strongest during the first five months after tetracycline came onto the market; after that, the effects leveled off. No particular group of doctors proved immune to the effects. Even the isolated doctors were influenced, although to a lesser extent than the integrated doctors and at a later point in time. Of the three types of social networks the sociologists studied—advisers, discussants, and friends—the strongest appeared to be the network of friends. That is, the largest effect appeared to come from informal discussions among doctors who socialized together.

Medical Innovation is often cited as a landmark study, and it is not hard to see why. It represents an enormous opportunity for drug marketers. Many of the ideas in both *Medical Innovation* and *Personal Influence* have become accepted as conventional marketing wisdom, especially the metaphor of communication as infectious disease. "Ideas and products and messages and behaviors spread like viruses do," writes Malcolm Gladwell in his influential book *The Tipping Point,* illustrating his argument with vivid stories of improbable social epidemics, from the vogue for Hush Puppies shoes among American hipsters to an outbreak of teen suicide in Micronesia.[14] *The Tipping Point* was an international best seller, and not merely by virtue of the ordinary nonfiction audience. Business readers transformed Gladwell into a fixture on the corporate lecture circuit.

While it makes a certain amount of sense that charismatic, socially connected experts would be better than most of us at transmitting messages, the evidence that things actually happen that way has been a little harder to verify. The Columbia University sociologist and Yahoo researcher Duncan Watts has tested the social contagion idea in a number of empirical studies and found that "influentials" are generally not that much better at transmitting word-of-mouth messages than the rest of us. "A rare bunch of cool people just don't have that power," he said in a 2008 magazine interview. "When you test the way marketers say the world works, it falls apart. There's no *there* there."[15] When marketers examine viral campaigns, they usually look at campaigns that have already been successful and then work backward, trying to identify the influential people who made them happen. But for every viral message that succeeds in starting an epidemic, there are many more that fail. If influentials are really so powerful, why do they fail so much more often than they succeed?

It may be that the particular circumstances surrounding a message are more important than the people transmitting it. For instance, tetracycline, the drug studied by the sociologists in *Medical Innovation,* was a very effective, easily administered antibiotic with few side effects.[16] It was aggressively promoted and competitively priced. These factors may well have been more important to its adoption than the social networking was. In fact, when the doctors in *Medical Innovation* were asked what sources of medical information they generally considered most important, they ranked the detail man far higher than they ranked their peers.

Are thought leaders really worth the money? The question is not that easy to answer. When a new drug is launched, it is promoted by such a variety of different methods, many of which straddle the gap between traditional mass-media marketing and peer-to-peer social networking, that it can be difficult to sort out just how much marketing success is due to which method. One study concluded that peer-to-peer networking resulted in an 11 percent greater likelihood over and above the pure marketing efforts that doctors would adopt a new drug.[17] Another study put the increased dollar value of peer-to-peer networking at just over 18 percent.[18] These studies indicate that thought leaders do have a significant effect, but it may be less than the hype suggests, and perhaps less than their compensation warrants.

• • •

What exactly do thought leaders do for companies when they are hired as consultants? The public got a rare glimpse in July 2009 when a committee of the U.S. Senate released the billing records of a prominent orthopedic surgeon. Dr. David Polly is chief of spine surgery at the University of Minnesota and a consultant to Medtronic, a Minnesota-based medical-device company. Polly made more than $1.14 million in consulting fees for Medtronic over a four-year period, an arrangement that prompted an anti-kickback lawsuit (which was later dismissed).[19] Polly's billing records were a model of efficiency and fine detail, logging his consulting services down to the minute. Some of the activities he billed Medtronic for were unsurprising, such as giving talks to colleagues and writing articles for publication. What caught the attention of the press was the expansive view Polly had of what counted as a consulting service.

For example, when Polly met with his local congressional representative to talk about the care of injured soldiers, he billed Medtronic $500. When he e-mailed with a local health insurer, he billed Medtronic $125. When he went to San Diego for a meeting of the North American Spine Society, he billed Medtronic $12,000—$4,000 for each day of the meeting. In 2006, the chief executive of Medtronic dropped in to the hospital to see Polly operate; Polly sent Medtronic a bill for $2,000. One morning in April 2006 Polly managed to make over $1,000 on the Medtronic expense account before seven a.m. To judge by the billing logs, every e-mail Polly answered, every phone call he returned, every meal he shared that could be connected to his surgical practice resulted in a charge to Medtronic at a rate of $500 per hour. Often these charges were logged in five-minute increments, each of which generated a fee of $49.48. At one point Polly even logged a one-minute wake-up call to a Medtronic executive, noting *no charge* for the call. However, he billed the company for the half hour he spent with the executive in the car later that morning.[20]

The most ill-advised service Polly provided to Medtronic came in May 2006, when Polly testified before a committee of the U.S. Senate.[21] Polly lobbied the Senate committee to fund research into spine and limb injuries suffered by American soldiers, telling the Senate that he was testifying on behalf of the American Academy of Orthopaedic Surgeons. What he did not tell the committee was that his trip was actually paid for by Medtronic, which manufactures Infuse, a bone-growth product used to treat such injuries. In total, Polly billed Medtronic more than $50,000 for costs related to political lobbying. Soon afterward, the U.S. Department of Defense awarded Polly and his colleagues at the University of Minnesota a $466,644 research grant to study Infuse.

What made Polly's failure to disclose his Medtronic ties to the U.S. Senate so spectacularly ill-advised was that for the past several years, Senator Charles Grassley, an Iowa Republican and the former chairman of the Senate Finance Committee, has made it his personal mission to investigate and expose the conflicts of interest generated when physicians work for the pharmaceutical and medical-device industry. When Grassley's staff investigates a potentially illicit financial relationship, it is generally not because of the relationship itself but the fact that the relationship has not been properly disclosed. Grassley's investigations have exposed ethically controversial practices in academic health centers such as Harvard, Stanford, and Emory. In July 2009, he sent a 142-page letter to the University of Minnesota documenting Polly's relationship with Medtronic and requesting its cooperation in the investigation.

Polly's Senate testimony may have been less prudent than usual, and his billing practices more detailed, but his financial relationship with Medtronic was far from the most egregious that Grassley has uncovered. In fact, part of the reason Grassley's investigations have continued to generate headlines—even in a post-Enron, post-Madoff era, where the public has become virtually numb to financial wrongdoing—is the sheer, unabashed bravado of the physician thought leaders he has investigated.

Not only do they appear outraged that they have been accused of wrong-doing, they often seem disdainful of any attempt to hold them account-able. Like the automaker CEOs who flew to Washington in corporate jets to ask for a government bailout, the thought leaders appear oblivious to the signals their behavior might send.

David Bronstein, the medical writer, refers to thought leadership as a cult, or maybe the priesthood. "At meetings they get big fancy badges, like generals with their medals," Bronstein says. They are given access to special VIP areas, where ordinary people cannot go. The thought lead-ers all know one another, because pharma companies introduce them. Aspiring young doctors cultivate relationships with thought leaders in order to advance their own careers.

Most drug reps, when pushed, can share stories about the arrogance of the thought leaders they were expected to flatter and serve. When Mi-chael Oldani was working for Pfizer, he used to deploy thought leaders regularly for dinner meetings and CME. Once he brought in a surgeon from Texas to talk about Diflucan. Oldani describes him as a "total ass." Oldani had organized a dinner meeting at a German restaurant, but the restaurant seated them in the basement, which was sweltering hot. "It's a sweat pit down there!" Oldani said to the manager, but there was no other place for them to go. The evening was a disaster. "A lady passed out into her strudel, facedown," says Oldani. "And it's an emergency, with an ambulance, and picture me: I'm like 'Christ, just throw some water on her and get her outside! She's ruining this program!'" The surgeon's talk was fragmented and disorganized, and when it finally ended, at ten p.m., Oldani was ready to go home and sleep. But the surgeon was not finished. "He tells me he needs some kind of alcohol to clean his mouse pad. And I'm like 'Really? I was just going to drop you off.' We drove around town for like an hour and a half until we finally found an all-night Walgreen's."

One of the most prominent thought leaders targeted by Senator Grassley's investigation was Dr. Charles Nemeroff, the former chairman of the Department of Psychiatry and Behavioral Sciences at Emory Uni-versity. Widely regarded as one of the most powerful psychiatrists in the country, Nemeroff has treated Atlanta luminaries such as Ted Turner, CNN leader Tom Johnson, and J. B. Fuqua, the businessman whose name graces the Fuqua School of Business at Duke. A psychiatry journal once referred to Nemeroff as the "boss of bosses." Another writer, less favor-ably disposed, gave him the nickname "Dr. Bling-Bling," referring to his ethically dubious financial relationships.[22] In 2002, Nemeroff published an article (without financial disclosure) in the journal *Nature Neurosci-*

ence praising three experimental psychiatric treatments from which he stood to profit, including a transdermal lithium patch for which he held the patent and from which he stood to gain as much as one million dollars in stock.[23] A few years later Nemeroff resigned as editor of the journal *Neuropsychopharmacology* after publishing one of his own coauthored articles praising vagal nerve stimulation, a treatment for depression that used a device manufactured by a company for which he was a consultant. In a memo to Nemeroff, a frustrated associate dean at Emory wrote, "I can't believe that anyone in the public or in academia would believe anything except that this paper was a piece of paid marketing."

Grassley's investigation found that Nemeroff had earned $2.8 million as an industry thought leader and researcher over a seven-year period and had failed to report $1.2 million. In 2004, Nemeroff signed a letter promising Emory officials that he would comply with federal rules and accept less than $10,000 annually from GlaxoSmithKline. But on the very day Nemeroff signed the letter, he checked into the Four Seasons Resort in Jackson Hole, Wyoming, courtesy of GlaxoSmithKline, which paid him $170,000 that year.[24]

Still, the most astonishing exchange to emerge from a Grassley investigation involved Dr. Joseph Biederman, a child psychiatrist at Harvard University who failed to report all but $200,000 of the $1.6 million in consulting fees he collected in an eight-year period. Biederman is probably the most prominent advocate of diagnosing bipolar disorder in children and treating it with antipsychotic drugs. One of those drugs (Risperdal) is manufactured by Johnson and Johnson, the company that underwrites the center that Biederman directs: the Johnson and Johnson Center for Pediatric Psychopathology Research at Massachusetts General Hospital. In a lawsuit against Johnson and Johnson, Biederman was accused of promising positive research results in exchange for funding.[25] A hint of Biederman's high self-opinion emerged in a deposition, where a lawyer asked Biederman about his academic ranking.[26]

BIEDERMAN: To move in the ranks from one rank, for example, at Harvard, there is instructor, from instructor you move to assistant professor, from assistant professor you move to associate professor, from associate professor you move to full professor.

LAWYER: Full professor?

BIEDERMAN: Mm-hmm.

LAWYER: What rank are you?

BIEDERMAN: Full professor.

LAWYER: What's after that?

BIEDERMAN: God.

LAWYER: Did you say *God*?

BIEDERMAN: Yeah.

• • •

Over the past several years some universities and professional organizations have begun to take action to mitigate the effects of payments to doctors. The most common solution is disclosure. Some states, such as Minnesota, have Sunshine laws, which require pharmaceutical companies to report payments to doctors. Grassley has cosponsored the Physician Payment Sunshine Act (PPSA), which would operate in a similar way. Disclosure of conflicts is usually presented as a win-win solution. Doctors get to keep accepting industry money; the drug companies get to keep giving it; and anyone else who might be affected can be reassured by the knowledge that the transactions are no longer secret.

Will strict disclosure rules solve the problem? "The funny thing about speakers is how many are not honest on their disclosure form," said Selina Mirza, a CME conference manager with the Texas Academy of Family Physicians, in an interview with *Medical Meetings* magazine. Leslie Ingraham of the University of New England agreed: "Short of reading a presenter's mind, we have very little to go on except what the speaker discloses to us."[27] These observations have been borne out by empirical research. Sheldon Krimsky of Tufts University has published a series of studies about disclosure in scientific and medical journals. One of those studies found that only 0.5 percent of over sixty thousand published articles in the scientific literature included any disclosure of competing financial interests. (In reality, an estimated quarter of those researchers probably had industry ties.) As Krimsky pointed out, those articles were published in high-impact journals that had clear guidelines on conflict of interest. At the time, most scientific journals did not even *ask* authors to disclose potential conflicts.[28]

It is not as if disclosure requirements would be a drastic change. Most journals and conferences now ask authors and speakers to disclose industry ties, and if not everyone complies, at least some do. Some states have had Sunshine laws for years. The main problem is not the failure to disclose but how empty the ritual of disclosure has become. Most disclosure statements are simply ignored, like the small print at the bottom of a rental-car agreement. Many KOLs even announce their industry relationships with something close to pride. (When a California psychiatrist was revealed as the top-earning thought leader for Eli Lilly in the first quarter of 2009, he replied that his patients approved of the industry payments. He lists his industry connections on his personal Web site.)[29] And why shouldn't KOLs be proud? If the reason academics work with industry is the status conferred by the relationship, then asking KOLs to reveal their industry ties is not that much different than asking them to reveal their honors and prizes.

The rationale for disclosure is the idea that transparency will eliminate—or at least minimize—the potential for bias. A physician with industry money can simply tell his audiences, patients, and research subjects up front what his financial interests are and let them make up their own minds what to do. In theory, this will minimize the effects of any bias that may have crept into the physician's decisions. Yet studies in psychology suggest that disclosure does just the reverse: it actually *increases* the potential for bias. The most interesting work on the topic has come from a group at Carnegie Mellon University. Their studies suggest that, far from remedying the bias created by conflicts of interest, disclosure may actually make the bias worse.[30]

The Carnegie Mellon group devised an experiment in which there were two groups of people, one called "estimators" and the other called "advisors." The estimators were instructed to stand off at a distance from large jars filled with coins and estimate how much money the jars had in them. The estimators were given a financial incentive to guess correctly. The closer the estimator came to guessing the right amount, the more money that particular estimator would get.

The other group, the advisors, had a different job and a different set of incentives. Their job was to stand much closer to the jars, look at the coins a lot more carefully, and then give written advice to the estimators. Unlike the estimators though, they were paid according to how high their estimators guessed. Their financial incentive was not based on how close to the truth their estimators got, but on how high their estimators' guesses were. In other words, they had a financial incentive to give misleading advice.

Some of the results were predictable. For example, when the estimators listened to the advisors, they made higher guesses. This is exactly what one would expect: after all, the advisors were getting paid to get the estimators to guess high. But another result was more surprising. When the advisors *disclosed* to the estimators that they were getting paid to have them guess high, the disclosure did not improve the estimators' guesses. That is, even though the estimators knew that the advisors were being paid to advise them to guess high, they continued to guess high. The fact that they heard a disclosure didn't make them any more skeptical of the advice they were getting.

A third finding was even more interesting. Once the advisors had disclosed their conflicts, their advice got worse. They began to give advice that was even more biased than before. It was as if the advisors had decided, *All bets are off now. I've disclosed my conflicts so now I'm free to say whatever I like.* The Carnegie Mellon group summed this finding up nicely when they said: Coming clean means playing dirty.

If the purpose of disclosure is to minimize the bias created by financial interests, then this research suggests disclosure may well be backfiring. But it also suggests that the effects of financial interests are more complex than we realize. As the Carnegie Mellon researchers point out, conflicts of interest are often not a problem of overt corruption or bribery. The people with conflicts are not intentionally misrepresenting the advice they give so that they will benefit financially. The bias in their advice is usually unconscious, which makes it especially difficult to remedy.[31]

•   •   •

David Healy is sitting across from me, working on a cup of bad coffee. We are at a table on the balcony of a hotel room in Scottsdale, Arizona, where Healy has just given a talk at the annual meeting of the American College of Neuropsychopharmacology (ACNP). It is December, but the day is warm enough for many people to be swimming in the outdoor pools. Healy is reminiscing about his days as an industry thought leader. "At one in the morning, I had an extremely attractive woman from Eli Lilly turn up at my bedroom door, scantily clad, with a tray of champagne, asking herself in," Healy tells me. Healy sent the woman away, but he says he cannot be sure about his colleagues. "I am absolutely certain from things I've been told that for opinion leaders in the field, services like this are laid on, if requested." As Healy thinks back to the old days he shakes his head, as if he can hardly believe what he used to get away with. "It's a glittering social thing," he says of industry events. "They hire the Opera House in Copenhagen for a meal. They hire the Metropolitan Museum of Art for a meal. If you were to ask my wife, she'd say: 'I miss the days when we'd fly into Geneva airport, and get picked up by a stretch limousine, and get driven to Montreux, and have the master bedroom in the Royal Hotel, overlooking the lake.' "

Healy is an academic psychiatrist, a historian of psychiatry, and a fierce critic of the pharmaceutical industry. For years he has appeared in the media arguing that the SSRI antidepressants such as Prozac, Zoloft, and Paxil can trigger suicidal thinking, and even suicidal acts. For an even longer period Healy has written on the risks of antidepressants, in the psychiatric literature and, perhaps most notably, in his book *Let Them Eat Prozac*. Healy's views have not made him popular with the pharmaceutical industry. Nor have they endeared him to his colleagues, most of whom do not share his worries about antidepressants. But it was not so long ago that Healy was an industry insider.[32]

Although Healy is Professor of Psychiatry at the University of Cardiff in Wales, he is an Irishman by birth. He grew up near Dublin, where his father was a civil servant in the health department, and he studied medicine at University College Dublin, from which he graduated with high honors in 1980. He went on to University College Galway, where he did a doctoral degree in neuroscience, and he trained in psychiatry at Galway, Dublin, and Cambridge. Healy was part of a new generation of biological psychiatrists coming into the field in the 1980s. By the early 1990s, when a number of antidepressants were being introduced, he had become secretary to the British Association for Psychopharmacology. "What happens when a drug like Prozac comes out is that they'll convene a bunch of senior academics," Healy says. "I ended up chairing meetings for an awful lot of the pharmaceutical companies."

The early 1990s saw the emergence of two competing narratives about the SSRI antidepressants. One was a "better than well" narrative. Many psychiatrists had noticed that the SSRIs did not help only those people who were clinically depressed. They also seemed to help some people with conditions that, by most definitions, did not count as any kind of mental disorder at all. Some clinicians called the drugs "mood brighteners," but it was psychiatrist Peter Kramer's term *cosmetic psychopharmacology* that caught on. In his book *Listening to Prozac*, Kramer worried about the consequences of using psychoactive drugs to make healthy people "better than well." According to this narrative, the primary ethical issue presented by the SSRIs concerned the use of prescription drugs to blunt the rough edges of ordinary life. Should doctors be prescribing psychoactive drugs to make healthy people cheerier, more energetic, and more outgoing?[33]

Competing with the "better than well" narrative was a much darker narrative about the side effects that the antidepressants could trigger. In 1990, Martin Teicher, a psychiatrist at Harvard University, published an article in the *American Journal of Psychiatry* outlining six case histories of patients who began having thoughts of suicide after taking Prozac (fluoxetine).[34] Teicher was not the only person who was worried. Similar stories were coming from patients themselves. Healy himself had two patients who had become suicidal on the drug. Soon Prozac was being featured on television and magazine news reports with headlines like "Prozac Backlash" and "Wonder Drug, Killer Drug." Healy asked representatives of Eli Lilly, the manufacturer of Prozac, what they thought about the suicide issue. "Help me out with this," Healy recalls asking Lilly. "What's going on? Have you seen this before?" Their response was: "Wouldn't you like to become a consultant to the company?"

Healy is a courtly, brown-haired man in his midfifties who bears a slight resemblance to the actor Gabriel Byrne. Cheerful and good-humored, he seems younger than his age, perhaps because he often seems on the verge of a smile. Healy has a slight stammer that often interrupts his speech, especially when he is nervous, yet he appears so accustomed to working around it that he barely even registers any self-consciousness. I have known Healy for about twelve years, mainly from academic conferences and a long-standing e-mail correspondence.

"Purely by chance, I was working on the serotonin reuptake system before any of the SSRIs had come on stream," Healy says. "And again, I was working on people who were depressed before it became highly fashionable for the industry to try to market mood disorders." Lilly began to invite Healy to meetings at a swanky hotel in the heart of London, where they would convene a dozen or so top psychiatrists. "You're thinking, you are in with the big guys now. And by the big guys, I don't mean industry. I mean you're in with senior figures in the field," Healy says. "These are the right people to know." Just as congenial as these senior figures were the company employees. "The people you will meet are often people who have moved over from medicine into industry, so they understand where you're coming from awfully well," says Healy. "It's not like the relationship between a salesman and you. You're dealing with people who went through the same system, who appear to have the same values, who could easily be in the same position you're in. They become your new best friends pretty quickly."

Healy also became familiar with public relations handlers and medical communications executives who managed and arranged his appearances at drug launches. "You meet a bunch of extremely attractive women who think what you have to say is great," Healy says. "And you have to go out for a meal with all the other people who are on the platform together—to bond, you know. You have to go to one of the best restaurants in town, of course, in Paris or Prague or Vienna. You meet to go over the slides." All the while you are managed by company handlers. "You have to get to the symposium, and you have to get to the press conference afterwards, so you get brought by your minders, your chaperones, from one to the other, and it feels good. You get brought through the crowd, the expert who has to be brought along to the next pressing engagement."

It is the glitter and flattery that Healy remembers most fondly from his industry days, not the intellectual life. "If you look at the opinion leaders, the guys in the field are not stellar geniuses," Healy says. "The field moves forward by virtue of the fact that people cooperate. It's not that anybody has a particularly brilliant insight, or that these guys are really awfully bright, but the opinion leaders who work with pharma are actually the *least* bright. They are the ones that it occurred to pretty early on that they're not going to get the chair at Harvard or Yale, but who do enjoy the lifestyle of being courted by industry, and having your articles written for you, of having articles in *JAMA* or *NEJM*, which you wouldn't otherwise have—these guys get made by industry. They get money, they get status, and they knew they wouldn't be anything if it weren't for this.

"We've moved from a world where there were comparatively few university people to a world where there are a load of them," says Healy. "And the industry can pick the people, based on their psychology and things like that, to suit their needs. They pick the kind of people who would like to have on their CV that they have written eight hundred articles. When in fact they have written ten or twenty, and the other seven hundred and ninety have been written by medical writers." Healy pauses and starts to grin. "There are people who you just see purr when the flattery comes in."

During the 1990s, Healy consulted for almost every major company with an interest in psychopharmacology. Yet at the same time, as an academic historian, he was writing critically about industry marketing. This criticism did not seem to bother his colleagues in the pharmaceutical industry. Nor were they especially upset by his views on the potential link between antidepressants and suicide. Healy says his industry colleagues seemed to think well of his 1997 book *The Antidepressant Era,* which was very critical of industry marketing practices but which gave the drug industry more credit than it had gotten in the standard "great man" histories that had preceded it.[35]

In 1998, Healy got a phone call from Baum Hedlund, a law firm in California that was interested in hiring him to do some legal work. Baum Hedlund was representing the family of William Forsyth in a lawsuit against Eli Lilly. Forsyth had been a prosperous businessman in his sixties when he retired to Hawaii. A psychiatrist gave him Prozac for anxiety. Forsyth had no history of violence and had never been hospitalized for depression in his life, yet eleven days after starting on Prozac, he stabbed his wife fifteen times and then fixed a kitchen knife to a chair and stabbed himself to death. Baum Hedlund wanted Healy to help them argue that Prozac had played a role.[36]

The question of whether the SSRIs can trigger suicide is difficult to parse. The difficulty comes from the fact that the condition the SSRIs are often prescribed to treat—clinical depression—is so closely associated with suicide itself. If a depressed patient commits suicide while on an SSRI, is it because of the drug or the illness? In fact, one of the dangers of an earlier generation of antidepressants, the tricyclics, is that they are dangerous in overdose. Psychiatrists are often reluctant to give patients too large a supply of tricyclics for fear they will kill themselves with the drugs. Yet there were signs from the start that the SSRI antidepressants were different. For one thing, clinicians had been reporting suicides of patients on SSRIs who were *not* depressed—who were taking the drugs for conditions that should not have increased their risk of suicide. One early series of case histories from Yale reported children becoming suicidal while being treated with SSRIs for obsessive-compulsive disorder.[37] There was also the weird association between SSRIs and violence. In the 1990s Lilly settled a lawsuit brought by the family of Joseph Wesbecker, a forty-seven-year-old man with a history of depression who, after starting Prozac in September of 1989, took an AK-47 to the printing press in Kentucky where he worked. He killed eight people and wounded twelve more before killing himself.[38]

Some psychiatrists believe that such suicides and homicides might be explained by a side effect of SSRIs termed *akathisia*. Akathisia is a kind of agitation and inner turmoil that ranges from restlessness and insomnia to extreme anxiety, bordering on panic. When German regulators rejected Lilly's application to market Prozac in Germany in the 1980s, they pointed especially to akathisia, saying that "an increase in agitating effects occurs earlier than mood-elevating effect and therefore an increased risk of suicide exists."[39] Of course, it was only on rare occasions that patients reacted this dramatically to SSRIs, suggesting that the drugs ordinarily were safe. Yet patients did need to be watched carefully, especially when they were starting the drug or discontinuing it, the times when the risk of suicide or violence was greatest.

When Healy was asked by Baum Hedlund to testify in the Forsyth case, he consulted with his industry colleagues. "What happens if I get involved in this?" Healy remembers asking. The lawsuits up until then mainly concerned Prozac, and Lilly's competitors did not seem to mind if he testified. Yet they did point out that testifying as an expert against the pharmaceutical industry was very rare. Healy remembers being told, "Mind you, this expert-witness stuff is the kind of thing that most people do toward the *end* of their careers. We're not quite sure why that is. But this is the way of the world."

Healy agreed to meet with Baum Hedlund, partly because AstraZeneca, a drug company for whom he was consulting, was flying him to a meeting taking place only about fifty miles from the Baum Hedlund office. After reviewing the Forsyth case, Healy agreed to testify. "The Forsyth trial was an extraordinary bunker-type thing," says Healy. "It is an intense emotional roller coaster. You have the trial team; they'll have a house; they'll have all the documents; they're trying to find a strategy; there are all the ups and downs of things that happen in court. And the whole thing will go on for a month or so." Taking part in a trial is very different from merely writing an expert report, says Healy. "If it gets to court, the whole thing is highly memorable. It's a little like being cornered by a rattlesnake."

As an expert witness against industry, Healy was granted access to internal information and study data that the public never saw. The more information Healy saw, the more he became convinced that the antidepressant manufacturers were hiding and manipulating studies in order to prevent the truth about the risks of antidepressants from coming out. "The fundamental issue here is that industry does not conform to the norms of science," he says. "They control the evidence completely. Industry now controls all the major journals in the field. They routinely get up and say, 'This is what the drug does.' And people don't even ask for the data, because they know they won't be shown the data."

The Forsyth case, like many others, was settled out of court. After his testimony against Lilly, however, Healy noticed that his career began to change.[40] Invitations to conferences stopped. Colleagues began to distance themselves. Healy found himself growing professionally isolated. In November 2000, Healy gave a lecture on the history of psychopharmacology at the University of Toronto's Centre for Addiction and Mental Health (CAMH), where he was scheduled to take up a new position as director of the mood disorders program. The position came with a large salary boost, as well as an increase in status: the University of Toronto is a large, internationally recognized research university with a distinguished medical school. In his lecture, Healy mentioned his worries about Prozac and suicide. Shortly thereafter, the CAMH rescinded his appointment. He was given no reason, merely informed by e-mail that CAMH did not feel that his "approach was compatible with the goals for development of the academic and clinical resource" of the clinic. CAMH officials later insisted that Eli Lilly had nothing to do with the decision, yet the CAMH had been a recent recipient of a $1.5 million gift from Lilly. The mood disorders program, which Healy was to direct, received 52 percent of its funding from corporate sources.[41]

The Toronto dismissal became an international academic scandal.[42] The Canadian Association of University Teachers backed Healy, as did a group of international figures in psychiatry and neuroscience, including two Nobel laureates. Although the University of Toronto was still reeling from a similar episode involving another dismissed faculty member, Nancy Olivieri, it refused to back down. Healy continued to speak out about antidepressants and the risk of suicide, and his dismissal became a flash point for larger political debates, not just about the potential dangers of antidepressants but also about financial conflicts of interest, whistle-blowers, and the influence of corporate money on academic medicine.

Yet Healy refused to behave the way that many of his supporters would have liked. He distanced himself from potential allies in the activist community by resisting any wholesale condemnation of the antidepressants, insisting that they were useful drugs if prescribed properly. He alienated those working to curb conflicts of interest by continuing to consult for the drug industry, including Pharmacia (now part of Pfizer), which had launched a new antidepressant called Edronax (reboxetine). He also decided to step up his work as an expert witness against the drug industry, making enemies of not just Eli Lilly but all the major antidepressant manufacturers.

Anyone who talks with Healy long enough about his troubles with the pharmaceutical industry will notice that, like Richard Nixon or Bob Dole, he slips easily into a habit of referring to himself in the third person. He talks about "the Healy problem," or "the rap on Healy," or how the drug industry failed to "kill off the Healy phenomenon." It is almost

as if he needs to separate his own identity from the picture of him created by the pharmaceutical industry, an image that emerged when he
began to testify against industry in court. "They didn't turn anti-Healy
on all this," he says, *this* referring to his written work. "The thing that
turned them anti-Healy was becoming an expert witness."

For several years, Healy was virtually alone, at least among medical-
establishment figures, in speaking out about the antidepressants' risk
of suicide. Although studies confirming his view began to mount in the
medical literature, most professional psychiatric organizations dug in
their heels on the side of the drug industry. Many warned that the suicide scare would frighten depressed patients from taking medication
for their illness and increase the rate of suicide. Healy became a target
for angry colleagues in the psychiatric community. A former friend in
Great Britain brought a complaint against him to the General Medical
Council, asking that his medical license be revoked. (The complaint was
dismissed.) A psychologist at the University of Pennsylvania published a
snarling essay in a bioethics journal about the sympathetic media treatment Healy had received, with the subtitle "The Martyrdom of David
Healy."[43]

Yet gradually, over a period of years, Healy has begun to see a measure of vindication. He filed a lawsuit against the University of Toronto
and the Centre for Addiction and Mental Health, seeking $9.4 million in
damages and lost income.[44] The case was settled out of court. While the
financial terms of the settlement were not disclosed, it was widely seen
as a victory for Healy. Conceding the damage to Healy's reputation, the
University of Toronto gave him a visiting professorship.

More significant has been a larger shift in opinion about the dangers of the antidepressants.[45] In June 2001, a Wyoming jury returned a
guilty verdict against GlaxoSmithKline, the manufacturer of the antidepressant Paxil, in a case where Healy had testified. The case concerned
a sixty-year-old man named Donald Schell who had gone to his doctor complaining of difficulty sleeping. He was given Paxil, and within
forty-eight hours, he killed his wife, daughter, infant granddaughter, and
himself. The jury awarded his surviving family $8 million.[46] Later, other
suicide cases began to attract media scrutiny. In 2004, the *New York
Times Magazine* published a lengthy article about the suicide of Matt
Miller, a thirteen-year-old boy who hung himself while taking Zoloft.[47]
In 2005, a healthy research subject, Tracy Johnson, committed suicide
in the Lilly research laboratory in Indianapolis while taking the antidepressant Cymbalta.[48]

Over the next several years, regulatory agencies and government bodies began to come around to Healy's views on suicide. The British government launched a parliamentary inquiry following a BBC documentary on the risks of Paxil, and in 2003, British regulators banned its use in children.[49] In 2004, GlaxoSmithKline, the manufacturer of Paxil, agreed to settle charges of consumer fraud for $2.5 million. The discovery process in that case revealed evidence that GlaxoSmithKline had deliberately suppressed unfavorable research about Paxil.[50] Later that year, the FDA reversed an earlier decision and placed a black-box warning on several SSRI antidepressants for patients under the age of twenty-five.[51]

Even so, Healy says he does not feel vindicated. "When you put forward the idea first, no one actually believes it," he says, shaking his head. "And then later on, when they do believe it, they say, 'Well, we've thought this all along, and you weren't the first to think of it—I was.'" Healy still feels the effects of his professional isolation. Many psychiatrists seem to blame Healy for making trouble but do not credit him for speaking out. "The average person does not thank you for pointing out that there is a shark in the water," Healy says. "The mayor wants to keep the beaches full. Don't tell anyone about the shark."

Healy still believes that academic physicians should work with the pharmaceutical industry, and that they should be paid for their work. Yet he does not think that most academic physicians appreciate the extent to which they are influenced. "Anyone who says to you that they are not conflicted by their ties to companies is lying, period," he says. "Anyone who says it doesn't have influence on them is lying. Anyone who says, 'Companies play me, but I play them,' and is convinced that they play companies to the same extent that companies are playing them, is lying. Or naïve." Yet Healy also has little patience with critics who insist that doctors should refuse to take any gifts or payments from industry. The real problem, he insists, is that the pharmaceutical industry controls the scientific evidence upon which medical practice is based. "Let me put it this way," he says. "It's an advantage for industry for you to think that the money is a problem. If every doctor in the world stopped getting money in the morning, stopped getting free pens, free lunches, trips to the Caribbean, and just went for the scientific evidence, we would have exactly the same problem as we have now." And that problem is the suppression and manipulation of scientific data.

Even to his admirers, Healy remains an enigmatic figure: a crusader against the drug industry who continues to accept industry funding; a pharmaceutical industry insider who works as a paid expert witness against industry. Healy insists that his view of the industry has remained essentially unchanged. "I haven't shifted at all," he says. "There has been no falling off the horse. I've had a slight double-agent streak the whole way through." Yet there is a problem with being a double agent that Healy does not seem to fully appreciate. A double agent is not fully trusted by either side, each of which suspects him of secretly working for the other.

•   •   •

In 1999 Merck launched its blockbuster pain drug the COX-2 inhibitor Vioxx. Within a year of its launch, prominent academic physicians, including Merck's own thought leaders, were raising questions about a possible link between Vioxx and heart disease.[52] Desperate to squelch this criticism, Merck executives began to circulate a list of thought leaders who needed to be "neutralized" or "discredited." In an internal e-mail, a Merck employee wrote, "We may need to seek them out and destroy them where they live."[53]

One such thought leader was Dr. Gurkirpal Singh, a rheumatologist with an adjunct appointment at Stanford University who had started to consult and speak for Merck in the late 1990s, nearly two years before Vioxx was launched. Merck had recruited Singh as a thought leader because of his research showing that naproxen, a competitor of Vioxx, was associated with gastrointestinal bleeding. Singh began giving grand-rounds lectures and dinner talks, commanding what a Merck salesperson described as "relatively large honoraria" of twenty-five hundred dollars per event. In a seven-month period, Singh gave forty talks for Merck.[54]

By early 2000, however, Merck had completed a large study that showed damaging results. The VIGOR study found that although Vioxx caused less gastrointestinal bleeding than naproxen, it was associated with an increased risk of heart disease. As Singh later told a Senate subcommittee, "The results of the VIGOR trial—a five hundred percent increase in the risk of heart attacks with Vioxx—stunned me. Clearly, the trade-off of five hundred percent increase in heart attacks for a fifty-percent reduction in stomach bleeds did not seem attractive." Merck duly submitted the VIGOR study to the FDA, but in the company's press releases, they gave the results a remarkable spin. Rather than concluding that Vioxx caused more heart attacks than naproxen, Merck claimed that naproxen *protected* the heart. Singh asked Merck repeatedly for the raw data from the VIGOR study. "I wanted to know how many heart attacks, how many strokes, how many deaths were occurring in each one of the groups, and what were these actual number of patients at risk, and how many ended up having an event." Merck stonewalled him, promising that the results would eventually be made public.

Frustrated with Merck's unresponsiveness, Singh began to speak openly about the potential risks of Vioxx. In his lectures he showed a cartoon of a man under a blanket, asking the audience to speculate about what Merck was hiding. At first, Merck responded by simply canceling Singh's lectures. But some people in the company worried that this strategy would backfire. An internal e-mail from a San Francisco–area business director said, "The one thing I am pretty sure of is that Dr. Singh could impact us negatively if he chose to do so . . . I would recommend we handle this very carefully . . . I just don't think canceling all the programs and walking away completely will serve us well in the long term."

Eventually, a senior executive at Merck, Dr. Louis Sherwood, made a telephone call to the home of a department chair at Stanford, Dr. James Fries, to inform him, as Fries later reported, that someone on his staff "had been making wild and irresponsible public statements about the cardiovascular side effects of Vioxx." Fries said that Sherwood hinted that if Singh did not stop his criticism, there would be repercussions for Fries. He was left with the impression that Merck's financial support of Stanford was in jeopardy. (In 2004, 9 percent of the Stanford medical school's research budget was supplied by the pharmaceutical industry.) Sherwood himself later explained the purpose of the phone call in an e-mail to a colleague. "Tell Singh that we've told his boss about his Merck-bashing. And tell him, should it continue, further actions will be necessary (don't define it)."

In the end, of course, Singh's suspicions about Vioxx were justified. Vioxx was eventually linked to an increased risk of heart disease and stroke. By the time Merck withdrew Vioxx from the market, in 2004, according to FDA reviewer David Graham, it had been responsible for over 38,000 deaths.[55] Merck eventually reached a $4.85 billion agreement to settle most of the personal-injury lawsuits over Vioxx.[56] The campaign to discredit Singh was not an isolated incident; Sherwood had made phone calls to a number of senior administrators at other medical schools and hospitals whose faculty members had been critical of Vioxx. Tom Nesi, a former pharmaceutical public relations executive who wrote a book about the Vioxx scandal, puts it this way: "They basically made up a hit list. They were sending this guy around, for lack of a better word, to shake people down."

How common are efforts by the industry to intimidate dissenters? It is hard to know, but only on rare occasions have efforts as overt as that of Merck been uncovered. "On the harassment front, pharma is usually more sophisticated," says Healy. "It's the things you expect to happen and don't that can drive you mad—the job offers, or invitations to speak, or promotions that don't happen." Many thought leaders who have clashed with pharmaceutical companies seem to regard the industry with such fear that companies do not really need to take any overt action to insure their compliance. Just a hint can be enough. Nesi says, "The amazing thing was how many people I spoke to who had dealt with the Merck people, the Pfizer people, the Monsanto people, the Searle people, who felt threatened—who felt that if they didn't go along with whatever study was coming out, that their careers would be jeopardized. Just about everybody I talked to said that."

Thought leaders and drug companies often approach one another with an attitude of congenial suspicion. Each party needs the other, but their interests often diverge. A thought leader must make a considered judgment about how trustworthy a company is, because he may find his credibility ruined if he promotes a drug that is dangerous or that has been marketed fraudulently. A company has to make a judgment about how much privileged information to reveal to its thought leaders, who not only have their own scholarly agendas but who may also be working for competing companies. If a thought leader turns on a company, the company may find its profits and reputation suffer. The delicacy of such arrangements means that collaboration involves a certain amount of calculation, like two seasoned poker players eyeing each other across the table, trying to figure out what cards the other is holding.

"There have been a lot of drugs that I have been involved with that have been taken off the market for one reason or another," says Daniel Metzger, the Ivy League gastroenterologist. Metzger is a man of good humor and strong opinions who cheerfully concedes that drug companies can be duplicitous. He worked with Merck on Vioxx and with Pfizer on its COX-2 inhibitors Bextra and Celebrex. "I was also a speaker for those companies, did CME programs, did a couple of visiting speakers' bureau programs on ulcer disease." He worked with Novartis on Zelnorm (tegaserod), a drug for irritable bowel syndrome that was removed from the market in 2007 after it was linked to a heightened risk of heart attacks and stroke. He worked with Janssen on Propulsid (cisapride), a drug that was used to treat heartburn until it was linked to heart arrhythmias. "Thank God I'm off that study," Metzger says. "I hated that study."

Metzger does not seem at all chastened by his experiences. "On the whole, I can't really say that I honestly regret the way I dealt with any of these," Metzger says. "I don't want to sound as if I think I am some sort of super-being here, but I can't think of any way that I have knowingly misinformed people." When the risk of heart disease and stroke with the COX-2 inhibitors became evident, Metzger says he began including information about those risks in his lectures. "The COX-2 inhibitors were a legitimate thing to investigate," he says. "I think the companies were a little unscrupulous, but I don't think my own involvement was in any way negative."

Metzger's attitude is not unusual. Nobody really seems to expect drug company executives to talk about potential problems with their drugs. Even drug reps rarely know in advance when a drug has serious problems. As one veteran drug rep, voicing a common sentiment, told me, "Reps are the last to know." Of course, a drug rep who details a drug enthusiastically right up to the day it is withdrawn from the market is likely to lose his or her credibility with doctors. Yet some reps say they don't hear about problems until the press gets wind of them and the company launches into damage control. At that point, Kathleen Slattery-Moschkau explains, "Reps learn verbatim how to handle the concern or objection in a way that spins it back in the drug's favor."

When a critic of a drug emerges, most companies understand that attempting to bully a critic into silence can easily backfire. It is much easier to blunt criticism by building alliances with your critics. "If I develop a contentious relationship with industry, I may actually get paid more," says Peter Whitehouse. "They might want to shut me up, or if they are smart, they may actually want to know what I am thinking. I may be able to help them more as a contrarian." (He adds that he is only speculating, and that he no longer accepts industry money.) David Healy, for all his disputes with the antidepressant manufacturers, does not seem inclined to cut his industry ties. "At this stage, I would have great market value for a pharmaceutical company," he says. "Especially if I were to come out and say, 'This is a great drug, and it's risk-free, it's actually going to work.'"

Many former thought leaders say that they get more criticism from their clinical colleagues than from industry. "Once you are an enemy of the people, you remain an enemy of the people," Healy says. Daniel Carlat, a Massachusetts psychiatrist, wrote regretfully about his work speaking on behalf of Wyeth in an article for the *New York Times Magazine* called "Dr. Drug Rep." It did not make him many friends in his field. "I am disliked by many prominent psychiatrists," he says. "Pariah is a strong word, but I'm on the edge of that category."

In any case, it is not always clear that coming out against a drug will damage its sales. It may simply make the name of a drug familiar to the public and help boost market share, especially in countries that do not allow direct-to-consumer advertising. Healy says that during the frenzied debate over a potential link between Prozac and suicide, he was approached by a public relations executive for Eli Lilly in the United Kingdom. "She actually came up to me and said, 'Oh, you're Dr. Healy. I'm so pleased to meet you. You're doing more for the sales of Prozac in this country than anyone else.' "

• • •

These days many thought leaders find themselves on shaky ground. The past few years have not been good for business. Some of the most prominent thought leaders have been exposed and censured by Grassley. Others have seen public opinion turning against them and gone underground. As more states institute Sunshine laws, anyone considering an industry consultancy must weigh the money and status boost against the potential downside of public exposure. Still, the thought-leader business has proved more resilient than many people predicted. Most of the thought leaders investigated by Grassley have managed to retain their academic positions, even in the face of withering criticism. A resistance movement has even formed. Led by Dr. Thomas Stossel of Harvard University, the Association of Clinical Researchers and Educators (ACRE) has defiantly opposed attempts to cut back industry payments to doctors.[57]

Many former thought leaders simply confess disillusionment. "There is a feeling that you want to be where the action is, and even if it's not real action, at least industry gives you the *feeling* that things are happening," Healy says. "They give you the feeling that you're up on the wave." After a while, however, the thrill of consulting begins to wear thin. There are just too many airports, too many hotels, too many fancy dinners. Eventually they all look the same. Healy says, "You've got a choice between the boredoms of perpetually surfing—where the first two waves are fun, but eight hours later, Jesus Christ—or do you return to the tedium of the beach?"

Carlat used to give talks on antidepressants but gave it up after deciding that he was being used as a marketing tool. Now he is an outspoken industry critic.[58] "The narcissistic satisfaction wears off, and then it is all about the money," he says. "You come to the realization that you're not being valued for anything important. You are valued for your commercial potential." At that point, a doctor has to decide whether it is still worth doing. Simply being the center of attention is enough to keep some of them on the lecture circuit. "Some people love to talk so much they never seem to get tired of it," Carlat says. "But it never gave me that much of a charge."

My brother Hal says the event that drove him away from his work for GlaxoSmithKline came when he was giving a lunch lecture at a local primary-care clinic. To his irritation, none of the doctors in attendance paid any attention to the lecture. They were answering pages, talking loudly to one another, helping themselves to the lunch that Glaxo had brought in—anything, it seemed, to avoid listening to him talk. Eventually Hal got so frustrated that he cut the lecture short. As he was packing up his laptop to leave, however, the Glaxo rep asked him a favor. The director of the clinic had been unable to attend the lecture. Would Hal mind sticking around a few more minutes to say hello? He would really appreciate it. Reluctantly Hal agreed, and the rep took him to a small room adjoining the clinic, where he said they would wait until the director appeared.

"There was a line on the floor," Hal says. He had never seen such a thing before. "The rep told me that we weren't supposed to step past that line unless the doctor said it was okay." They stood behind the line, waiting patiently. After a few minutes, the director walked down the hall toward them. "I sort of looked at him, hoping to make eye contact and speak, but he wouldn't even look at us," Hal says. "This rep just stood there with a big smile on his face, and the doctor stopped in front of the treatment room five feet away from us, and stood there for several minutes reading a chart. Then he walked away into the treatment room like we were not even there."

Hal calls this his moment of understanding, after which he never gave another industry-funded talk. Up to that point, he had imagined himself as a high-powered academic physician bringing the latest university research to doctors out in the community. Standing next to the drug rep, however, Hal understood how the community doctors saw him. To them, Hal was a drug company shill. "I was literally standing in the drug rep spot begging for a minute of this doctor's time, like a cocker spaniel begging for a leftover piece of meat from the table," he says. It was no wonder the doctors saw little difference between Hal and the rep. "It was like I had become a psychiatric callboy," he says. "I might as well have just said, 'Hi, I'm Hal. The company sent me to make sure you all have a good time.'"

CHAPTER FIVE

The Flacks

SEVERAL YEARS AGO, I was sitting in my office at the University of Minnesota trying to avoid work when I got an unusual phone call. It came from an international advertising agency. The woman on the phone said she had read my book *Better than Well* and wondered if I would talk about it at a meeting in Boston. I had no idea what to make of her invitation. It was hard for me to imagine why anyone in an advertising agency would want to hear about my book, which was not exactly enthusiastic about the marketing business; besides, this company did not even seem to market drugs. They advertised consumer products such as cars, bourbon whiskey, and golf balls. Out of curiosity, I agreed to go.[1]

The meeting was for the company's strategic planners, who had been flown to Boston from various international locations. Strategic planners, I learned, are hip young people who dress in black and wear small, stylish glasses. In the advertising world, their job description appears to fall somewhere between "ethnographer" and "evil genius." Unlike the "creatives," who were not present at the meeting but who were often invoked, like mysterious spirits, strategic planners do not actually create ads. They are the intellectuals behind the operation. It is part of their job to hit the streets, sniff the air, and figure out what can be exploited for capitalism. These strategic planners had gathered in Boston to brainstorm about their various marketing campaigns, one of which concerned a new Volkswagen.

The Volkswagen campaign was tricky. Volkswagen was producing a luxury car called the Phaeton, which it planned to price at over $70,000 (and which actually wound up costing much more). Volkswagen envisioned the Phaeton as an elite, high-end competitor to Jaguar, BMW, and Mercedes. For the strategic planners, the problem with the Phaeton was the Volkswagen brand. Volkswagens are not exactly branded for luxury. If anything, they are branded with a kind of hip nostalgia for the 1960s counterculture. So the strategic planners had a dilemma. To sell a luxury car like the Phaeton, they had to reach luxury-car buyers. But they did not want to alienate the Volkswagen brand loyalists. How do you sell luxury Volkswagens without looking like a sellout to all those guys in denim jackets and gray ponytails who associate Volkswagens with the smell of weed and the sound of the Grateful Dead?

After months of research, the strategic planners had constructed a detailed approach. To sell luxury Volkswagens, they believed, you need to find a particular kind of customer. Ideally, these customers are creative, environmentally sensitive liberals who are concerned about social justice. They are the sort of people who read the *New York Times,* listen to National Public Radio, and shop at Whole Foods. They spend a lot of time in coffee shops and bookstores, and they are closely involved with their neighborhood organizations and their children's schools. And of course, their stock portfolios are impressive enough for them to drop $70,000 on a luxury car.

Unfortunately, however, there is a problem with this particular psychographic. These people are deeply cynical about advertising. Only rarely do they watch television, and when they do, they filter out all the ads with TiVo. So how do you market to them? Here is where I began to grasp the dark allure of strategic planning. The planners were going to find out what left-wing charities their customers favored, where their kids went to school, and what neighborhood organizations they were involved in. Then they planned to donate money to those groups and make sure everyone knew about it as a way to generate word-of-mouth buzz. My host at the meeting, a former literature professor who now worked as a "cultural strategist" for the company, was practically rubbing his hands with delight. He kept leaning over to me and whispering things like "So what would Marx think about this one, eh?" and "Talk about seizing the means of production!" My role in this meeting was to talk briefly about my book as a kind of light entertainment for the strategic planners while they plotted how to sell cars.

As ingenious as the plan was, it appears to have backfired spectacularly. When the Phaeton was introduced to the United States, the *New York Times* featured an article about it headlined "A People's Car for Wealthy People."[2] In 2004 only 1,433 of these cars were sold, and when sales dropped the next year to a mere 820, Volkswagen announced that the Phaeton would be discontinued.[3] (It was later reintroduced.) It is hard to know whether these disappointing sales were a result of an ill-conceived marketing campaign or if the problem was the Phaeton itself. However, the difficulty marketing the Phaeton is symptomatic of a deeper predicament facing any advertising agency today. How do you market a product to customers who are thoroughly contemptuous of advertising?

Drug marketers have faced this problem for years. Prescription drugs are bought and sold as market commodities, but nobody is entirely comfortable thinking of them as a consumer good. Prescribing decisions are supposed to be made on the basis of scientific evidence, not whim or preference; the decision-makers are highly educated professionals who are meant to put the patients' interests first, and the stakes involved in a single prescription can be alarmingly high. Few of us are unreservedly enthusiastic about inserting pharmaceutical sales into the machinery of consumer capitalism, at least when one's individual health is on the line. It would be as if the NASA engineers decided which materials to use for the space shuttle based on which company had produced the cleverest television ads.

For the psychic comfort of everyone involved, drug marketing needs to be disguised. Developing this disguise is the job of public relations. The public relations specialist does not market a product so much as he or she manipulates conditions in such a way that more of the product is sold. The manipulation must be accomplished subtly and carefully, without calling too much attention to itself, for if the disguise falls off, the campaign will fail. Yet the covert nature of public relations makes the manipulation feel especially fraught. You organize a charity event, but your real purpose is to publicize a drug. You pitch a news story about the new consumer trend for eco-friendly living, but your real aim is to market a new hybrid car. Gradually, you begin to see all the things of ordinary life as potential marketing devices. This kind of marketing is uncomfortable in a creepy new way. News, conversation, friends, humanitarian aid: virtually anything can be used as a sales instrument, but one that's effective only as long as nobody realizes that a product is being sold.

Shortly after my Boston meeting, I came across a book by Al Ries called *The Fall of Advertising and the Rise of PR.*[4] Ries, a former adman, lists a string of successful companies, from Starbucks and the Body Shop to Amazon and Intel, that built their brands almost entirely without advertising. "We have seen the future of marketing," Ries said in a 2004 lecture in New York.[5] "The future of marketing is Botox." The audience laughed, but Ries was not joking. When Allergan introduced Botox in 1993, Ries said, the drug generated $25 million in sales. Yet by 2001, Botox was generating $300 million in sales. How did Allergan manage an elevenfold increase in sales in only eight years? "No advertising, no advertising, no advertising, no direct mail," Ries said. "No nothing but PR."

Suppose you were offered a choice, says Ries. A magazine will give you a free advertisement, or they will run your story as an article. "How many companies would prefer an ad to an article?" Ries asks. "No one. Advertising has no credibility."[6] But many people still believe what they read in magazines. It is this credibility that public relations exploits. The public relations expert is always asking himself: How do I take the credibility of a trusted authority and use it for my own purposes?

• • •

Stacy Carter got involved with the anti-smoking movement when she was working on her graduate degree in public health. Her mentor was an anti-smoking activist as well as an internationally recognized academic researcher at the University of Sydney. Carter went to work for him as a research assistant for a smoking-cessation project. Her job was to produce an anti-smoking monograph called "Finding the Strength to Kill Your Best Friend"—a title that seems slightly alarming until you realize that a smoker's best friend is supposed to be his cigarette habit.

Carter is a tall, slender Australian in her late thirties with an easy laugh and the look of an athlete. Before she went into public health, Carter worked for six years as a speech pathologist for stroke patients. She has a genuine, open manner that puts people at ease. When "Finding the Strength to Kill Your Best Friend" was complete, Carter was selected as the media spokesperson for the project. "I'm not sure why they picked me to be the talking head," she says, wondering aloud if the company needed a woman or if it was simply that no one else wanted the job. "Somehow I ended up being the bunny." For a week or so Carter answered phone calls from journalists and explained the findings of the project. All the media attention was flattering. The public relations specialist told her she was a natural.

One day Carter was scheduled for a video shoot with Palin Communications, a health-care public relations company based near Sydney. At the beginning of the shoot, a production assistant put a hand on Carter and told her, "You're going to be a star today, my dear." First came a question-and-answer session in Carter's office. Then the company filmed some footage of Carter and her mentor strolling through the grassy sandstone quadrangle at Sydney University, pretending to have a learned conversation. When Carter saw the finished video a few weeks later, however, she was surprised. It looked like a news segment intended for distribution to television news stations. The narrative centered on a famous rugby player who had quit smoking. It also included a number of features apparently meant to disguise the fact that the news station had not produced the video, such as a script for local television reporters to read. "My comments were preceded by blank spaces into which the journalists could insert their questions," she says. Also helpfully provided were the questions themselves.

In the public relations business, such productions are known as video news releases, or VNRs. A VNR is a simulated news story designed to be indistinguishable from ordinary television news. Its purpose is to generate publicity for an idea or a product, often with the aim of selling it. Some VNRs are commissioned by government agencies and nonprofit groups, but most are commissioned by corporations. The funding for the VNR in which Carter appeared came from the pharmaceutical company GlaxoSmithKline, which manufactures nicotine-replacement therapy and the smoking-cessation drug Zyban. Critics call VNRs fake news, but Carter says she did not find her VNR particularly objectionable, at least not right away.[7] "I was not horrified," she says. "At the time, I thought: so that's how it works."

According to public relations specialists, VNRs are simply the television equivalent of a press release. They have been around for about forty years. Television stations began using VNRs more widely in the 1980s, when local budgets began to drop and stations needed an inexpensive way to fill airtime. Eventually, VNRs became a popular way for pharmaceutical companies to generate coverage of new drugs.[8] Some VNRs are broadcast on the news unedited, with commentary and narration provided by the company, while others feature raw footage known as B-roll, which can be edited by local stations. Some surveys have found that over 90 percent of U.S. television stations broadcast VNRs.[9] When Pfizer launched Viagra in 1998, for example, a single VNR on the drug was seen by more than a hundred million people.[10]

"Our job is to make it look, feel, sound, smell, and taste like news," says Michael Friedman. Friedman is a silver-haired, disarmingly blunt senior executive at DWJ Television, a New Jersey–based company that has produced over thirty thousand VNRs since the 1970s. Friedman starts by getting as much information as possible about a product. "We'll put it into television language and come up with a script that runs about ninety seconds," he says. When the VNR is complete, the placement department will start pitching it to televisions stations. If thirty-five to fifty stations broadcast the VNR, it is considered a success.

Production companies often build VNRs around events that are manufactured or exaggerated for dramatic purposes. For pharmaceutical VNRs, the most convenient event is the approval of a new drug by the FDA. But sometimes a production company has to get more creative. "If there is no hard news, we will generally do it in terms of a disease, and get a real person suffering from the condition who has had it improved by taking this medication," Friedman says. "So we may see him or her with a physician; we may see him or her doing things in everyday life; and we'll also interview on-screen, and interview the physician on-screen." Many production companies build VNRs around disease-awareness events. The National Sleep Foundation, an organization funded by manufacturers of sleep drugs and other sleep aids, often uses National Sleep Awareness Week as a hook, usually coupled with a survey about how much trouble Americans have sleeping. "To me, that's the last possibility," says Friedman. "There's always a day, there's always a week, there's always a month. The only one that resonates is Breast Cancer Awareness Month. Everybody goes gangbusters on that. But, you know, heart month, none of those really do much for me."

Another popular hook is a relevant social trend. When DWJ needed to come up with a VNR for Singulair, an asthma drug produced by Merck, the company took advantage of the widespread public concern about the prevalence of asthma. "We must have done about eight VNRs on that, starting with the FDA approval. We did allergies and asthma; we did cold-weather asthma; we did warm-weather asthma; we did inner-city asthma. It was the same solution, but a different problem," says Friedman. "We just rode that tide." That strategy worked for nearly two years.

VNRs are only one of many broadcasting tools produced by DWJ. Among the video samples included on their Web site is a clip featuring the actress and dancer Rita Moreno.[11] As a doctor fingers a plastic replica of the human spine, Moreno says, "I never thought that osteoporosis would affect me. My doctor says that because I am past menopause, I should have a bone density test along with a mammogram and other health-care screenings." As Moreno eases herself onto an examining table, she reassures the viewer: "The bone density test was quick, easy, and painless."

The video clip is a PSA, or public-service announcement. A PSA is a short segment television and radio stations run between regular programs, like advertisements, that's intended to change public attitudes about a specific issue. Perhaps the most famous PSA is the "This is your brain on drugs" spots sponsored by the Partnership for a Drug-Free America in the 1980s. (Ominous music broadcast during footage of a frying pan with oil. "This is drugs," says a deep, gravelly voice. An egg drops in and starts to fry. "This is your brain on drugs. Any questions?") Most PSAs concern issues of health or safety—just say no to drugs, don't drive drunk, please fasten your seat belt. Although some PSAs are sponsored by nonprofit groups, many are backed by corporations. A pharmaceutical industry–backed PSA might ask you to get a flu shot, have your cholesterol checked, or undergo screening for Alzheimer's disease.

The great advantage of PSAs is their low cost. DWJ can produce a television PSA for $35,000 to $50,000, and a radio PSA costs a mere $13,000 to $20,000. And unlike advertisements, which may cost millions to place on television, PSAs are broadcast for free. They are considered a noncommercial civic good, like children's shows or community broadcasting. The disadvantage is that the sponsor cannot schedule PSAs at a specific time, or even be sure they will be aired. Those decisions are up to the station. Broadcasters typically use PSAs to fill up airtime that has not sold to commercial sponsors.

Of course, the entire rationale for broadcasting PSAs, as the name suggests, is that they are a public service. And if the sponsor of a PSA is a commercial organization that aims to generate sales for a product, the commercial sponsorship needs to be downplayed—not just in the PSA itself, but in the cover letters that are sent out to broadcasters. On its Web site, DWJ advises people writing letters on behalf of sponsors to avoid identifying themselves as brand marketing and advertising managers and instead use titles such as public-service advertising managers and public education managers.[12] The letters should also avoid commercial language. DWJ advises, "The sponsoring organization, in whose name the spots are presented, ideally should be a nonprofit organization as defined by section 501(c)(3) of the IRS code."

The ingenuity of PSAs is not simply that they hide a commercial message behind a façade of civic responsibility. It is that they are often aimed at genuinely admirable goals. When Stacy Carter looks back at her unknowing public relations efforts on behalf of the GlaxoSmithKline smoking-cessation campaign, knowing now that their real aim was to promote Zyban, it is not entirely with regret. Her VNR may well have helped convince some viewers to stop smoking. She says, "I don't think it did a great deal of harm, and it may have done some people good."

What Carter does regret is her own naïveté. She was so caught up in the moral crusade against cigarettes that she did not notice that the crusade was backed by a pharmaceutical company with its own commercial interests. It was only when Carter began to do research on access to drugs in the developing world that she came to understand how deftly the pharmaceutical industry had used her. "I started to feel ashamed that I could have been duped so easily," she says, marveling at how mechanically she followed the script. "I was a pawn in this pharmaceutical industry game, without ever being told what to do."

The VNR may soon be a relic of the past. According to Michael Friedman, the demand for VNRs has died away. Friedman blames an activist campaign by the Center for Media and Democracy, a small, persistent nonprofit group in Madison, Wisconsin. "They killed the VNR," says Friedman. "The only time I can do a VNR now is for an FDA approval, and if I have a celebrity. Aside from that? Dead." Instead, Friedman now produces satellite media tours. He hires experts to come into the studio for interviews, mainly on the morning talk shows, that are broadcast live through satellite video links. He provides the interviewers with questions to ask and trains the experts to deliver a PR message in as little as fifteen seconds. The expert spends the morning doing back-to-back interviews with one talk show after another. "The spots usually last about two and a half minutes," Friedman says. "We work for four hours and do about twenty to twenty-five comfortably. At the end of four hours the person is drained, I assure you."

• • •

In 1922, a controversial play called *Damaged Goods* was about to open in New York.[13] The play was about syphilis. Written by Eugene Brieux, a French playwright, *Damaged Goods* concerned a young man with syphilis who, against the advice of his physician, got married. Soon he and his wife produced a syphilitic child. The play was pure melodrama, but its message lined up squarely with the aim of public health: to get the topic of venereal disease into public view, where it could be discussed openly and prevented. The problem was that the New York Society for the Suppression of Vice had closed down other plays that it had deemed too daring for the time, and the group had the backing of the police and the mayor. The producer of *Damaged Goods* feared that his play would be closed down as well.

The problem facing *Damaged Goods* came to the attention of a young man named Edward Bernays, a Cornell graduate who was editing two medical publications, *Dietetic and Hygienic Gazette* and *Medical Review of Reviews*. Intrigued by the play, Bernays orchestrated a series of behind-the-scenes actions designed to ease it into public acceptance. He began by establishing an apparently independent third party called the *Medical Review of Reviews* Sociological Fund Committee. The objective of the committee was to educate the public about venereal disease. Bernays rounded up backers from the upper strata of New York society— a Rockefeller, a Vanderbilt, a Flexner, and others—by appealing to their enlightened attitudes. "I was careful to invite men and women whose good faith was beyond question and would be responsive to our cause," Bernays later recollected.[14] Only after the *Medical Review of Reviews* Sociological Fund Committee was up and running did Bernays announce its first project: to back the production of *Damaged Goods*. His plan worked perfectly. *Damaged Goods* opened to enthusiastic reviews and was heralded as a tool of public enlightenment. Woodrow Wilson came to a special performance. A touring company was formed, and the play was taken on the road.

Perhaps the most lasting result of *Damaged Goods*, however, was its guiding Edward Bernays to his true vocation: public relations. By the time he died, in 1995, at the age of 104, Bernays had spent nearly three quarters of a century writing books on PR strategy and designing campaigns for products, charities, and political causes. Bernays polished the images of John D. Rockefeller and Calvin Coolidge; he persuaded a generation of American women to begin smoking cigarettes; he even helped the U.S. government and the United Fruit Company overthrow the democratically elected president of Guatemala. He also changed the nature of publicity. Press agents had traditionally generated news coverage simply by handing out press releases and staging press conferences. Bernays had far greater ambitions. He envisioned a professional "public relations counsel" secretly pulling the levers of power, manipulating figures as if on a chessboard without their conscious awareness. Today Bernays is remembered not merely as an influential practitioner of public relations but as the most important intellectual behind the movement.[15]

Bernays saw the news the way a choreographer sees a stage. "Newsworthy events, involving people, usually do not happen by accident," Bernays wrote. "They are planned deliberately to accomplish a purpose, to influence our ideas and actions."[16] With the right script, set, and cast of characters, the public relations expert could take control of the news, orchestrating "spontaneous" events that would lead the public to perceive the world in a certain way. In the 1920s, for instance, Bernays sent out a group of models to march in a New York City parade while smoking cigarettes ("torches of freedom," Bernays called them), ostensibly to protest against the taboo against women smoking in public. The *New York Times* reported the event with the headline: "Group of Girls Puff at Cigarettes as a Gesture of Freedom." In fact, the purpose of the demonstration was to promote cigarette sales for the American Tobacco Company.[17] Bernays summed up his vision of public relations in heroic terms: "When Napoleon said, 'Circumstance? I make circumstance,' he expressed very nearly the spirit of the public relations counsel's work."[18]

For Bernays, people were creatures of psychological habit that could be swayed by appeals to the "herd instinct." As he wrote in his 1928 book *Propaganda,* "If we understand the mechanism and motives of the group mind, is it not possible to control and regiment the masses according to their will without their knowing it?"[19] A nephew of Sigmund Freud and an avid student of his ideas, Bernays saw people as slaves to their unconscious instincts and desires.[20] Unlike Freud, however, who used the techniques of psychology to open up the unconscious mind, Bernays used them to keep the unconscious hidden.[21] Most people do not really understand why they buy the things they buy or hold the opinions they hold, he believed, and this lack of understanding could be exploited. If the public relations counsel can just pull the right strings, he can make people dance like puppets.

If this sounds menacing and overblown, like the boasts of a comic-book villain, it is partly because Bernays was such an active propagandist on his own behalf. He spent decades polishing his own reputation as a sage and crafty influence broker. Yet Bernays really was an old-school elitist, a true believer in the ruling class. He was convinced that democracy could work only if it were guided by a seasoned, managerial aristocracy. It was no stretch for him to position himself as an intellectual mastermind pushing the buttons that make the robots lurch forward because he genuinely thought of himself that way. In *Propaganda,* he portrays the public relations counsel as a detached professional, one of the "invisible governors" who coolly observe and manipulate the receptive, unthinking masses. He wrote, "It is they who pull the wires which control the public mind, who harness old social forces and contrive new ways to bind and guide the world."[22]

The term *invisible governors* would turn out to be prophetic. Today the average American probably cannot name a single public relations company or even say what they do, yet the techniques of public relations permeate the culture in a way that is hard to exaggerate. We live in a political landscape filled with lobby groups and public-opinion pollsters. The corporate world is dominated by multinational public relations companies such as Weber Shandwick, Hill and Knowlton, Ketchum, and Burson-Marsteller. No company, university, or government body of any size would be without a communications office, whose job is to protect the interests and reputation of its employer. The elitist vision of Bernays has gone out of fashion, but marketers and politicians have embraced the tactics he developed. Unlike many traditional marketers, however, who must dance frantically in the spotlight to sell their products, the public relations expert watches silently from the wings.

Bernays mastered the art of selling without the appearance of salesmanship. It was his gift to see how social conditions could be manipulated in order to increase sales in ways that were invisible to the customer. When Bernays worked on behalf of Mozart pianos, for example, he did not simply recommend the piano on its merits; he promoted the idea of the music room in the home. By making the music room a mark of sophistication, something that no educated, well-heeled American could afford to be without, Bernays did not so much sell pianos as create the conditions for the pianos to sell themselves. "And the man or woman who has a music room, or who has arranged a corner of the parlor as a musical corner, will naturally think of buying a piano," Bernays wrote. "It will come to him as his own idea."[23]

•   •   •

Many of us have a relatively simple, commonsense view of the way that drug development and marketing work. People get diseases; scientists develop drugs to treat those diseases; and marketers sell the drugs by showing that the drugs work better than their competitors. Sometimes, however, this pattern works in reverse. Drug company scientists develop a drug with a range of physiological effects, none of which are terribly helpful, so the marketers must identify and promote a disease for the drug to treat. This might mean co-opting a rare disease whose borders can be expanded to encompass more patients, or redefining an unpleasant aspect of ordinary life as a medical pathology. Once a disease has achieved a critical degree of cultural legitimacy, there is no need to convince anyone that a drug is necessary. It will come to him as his own idea.

A classic drug industry example is the strategy developed by Merck in the 1960s to promote amitriptyline, its new antidepressant. At the time, clinical depression was regarded as a rare condition—so rare, in fact, that there appeared to be little profit in marketing an antidepressant. The solution was to increase the frequency of the diagnosis. To that end, Merck bought fifty thousand copies of a book by Frank Ayd called *Recognizing the Depressed Patient* and sent them out free of charge to general practitioners all over the country. Prescriptions for amitriptyline took off dramatically, despite the fact that a similar antidepressant, imipramine, had been available since the mid-1950s. The key to selling antidepressants, it became clear, was to sell clinical depression.[24]

Fifty years ago this kind of marketing was aimed mainly at doctors. Today it is also directed at patients. The marketing buzzword is *disease branding*.[25] To brand a disease is to shape its public perception in order to make it more palatable to potential patients. This is usually done by telling people that the disease is taken seriously by doctors, that it is far more common than they ever realized, and that having it is nothing to be ashamed of. As Vince Parry, the president of Y Brand, puts it, disease branding is a "win-win marketing strategy that illuminates, educates and promotes at the same time."[26]

Disease branding works especially well for two sorts of conditions. The first is the condition that, like clinical depression in the early 1960s, can be plausibly portrayed as common yet underdiagnosed. This sort of branding campaign legitimates the pain or discomfort that people experience, not just by giving it a clinical name but by assuring potential patients they are part of a large community of sufferers. Take, for instance, restless legs syndrome. Until recently, restless legs syndrome was seen by clinicians as an unusual, somewhat mysterious condition. It was characterized by a crawling or aching sensation in the legs, often more severe at night, which could be relieved by movement such as walking. It was not a common affliction. In 2005, however, GlaxoSmithKline got approval from the FDA to market Requip, a drug used to treat Parkinson's disease, as a treatment for restless legs syndrome. GlaxoSmithKline soon issued a press release titled "New Survey Reveals Common Yet Under-Recognized Disorder—Restless Legs Syndrome—Is Keeping Americans Awake at Night." The Requip public relations campaign went on to suggest that problems such as insomnia and depression might actually be symptoms of restless legs syndrome, which tormented as many as one in ten Americans.[27]

The second disease-branding candidate is the shameful condition that can be destigmatized. When Pharmacia launched Detrol in late

1990s, for instance, the condition it treated was known to doctors as *urge incontinence*. Patients called it "accidentally peeing in my pants," and they were reluctant to mention it to their physicians. Pharmacia responded by rebranding *urge incontinence* as *overactive bladder*. This helped in two ways. First, whereas *urge incontinence* implied a kind of constitutional weakness and was associated mainly with elderly people, *overactive bladder* suggested that patients were afflicted by some sort of supercharged organ frantically working overtime. This shift from weakness to strength made the condition seem less embarrassing. Second, in contrast to *incontinence,* which meant actual loss of bladder control, *overactive bladder* was defined to include people who very often simply had a strong urge to go to the bathroom. The vice president of Pharmacia, Neil Wolf, explained his strategy in a 2002 presentation called "Positioning Detrol: Creating a Disease." By creating the disease of overactive bladder, Wolf said, Pharmacia expanded the treatable population nearly threefold, to a total of twenty-one million potential patients—the difference between a "niche product" and a "mass-market opportunity." By 2003, Detrol and its long-acting version, Detrol LA, accounted for $757 million in annual sales.[28]

Because it is difficult to create a disease without the help of physicians, companies typically recruit physician thought leaders to write and speak about any new concepts they are trying to introduce. "It is always presented as a scientific and clinical opportunity to help patients," says Peter Whitehouse, a neurologist at Case Western Reserve University. Physicians must be convinced that a new disease category actually describes a patient population whose symptoms warrant a drug. It also helps if the physicians believe the condition is dangerous. When AstraZeneca introduced Prilosec (and later Nexium) for heartburn, for example, it famously repositioned heartburn as gastroesophageal reflux disease, or GERD. But it also commissioned research to demonstrate the devastating consequences of failing to treat it.[29] Once physicians are on board, a company can get a concept like overactive bladder or reflux disease into widespread circulation simply by funding CME events, journal supplements, and disease-awareness campaigns. "That's easy," says Whitehouse. "You just have to have enough money."

If a marketing campaign is really successful, it goes beyond hype to insinuate itself into the language and thought of the population as a whole, essentially remaking the way people think of themselves. Concepts such as reflux disease, erectile dysfunction, and irritable bowel syndrome have had considerable success, but the most remarkable changes have come in the language of psychiatry with the emergence of neurobiological concepts such as social anxiety disorder, attention deficit hyperactivity disorder, and bipolar disorder. What is striking about this neurobiological language is the extent to which ordinary people have come to incorporate it into their identities. You may *have* erectile dysfunction or irritable bowel syndrome, but you *are* bipolar or ADHD. Your diagnosis is part of who you are.[30]

In some ways, these changes simply reflect the transformation of psychiatry into a biological discipline. Just as terms such as *repression* and *inferiority complex* moved from the specialized world of psychotherapy out into the culture as a whole in the mid-twentieth century, these neurobiological concepts have migrated out of biological psychiatry into more common use. In earlier times the paradigm was the language of unconscious conflicts; now, it is the language of neural circuits, molecular genetics, and brain imaging. Yet these neurobiological concepts go even further than those they have replaced. They introduce new ways to be a human being. The bipolar child, the socially anxious adult, and the ADHD student did not exist thirty years ago, at least not in the modern way. They have emerged in response to medication.

This is not an unprecedented phenomenon. As the philosopher Ian Hacking has explained, new identities have often arisen in different historical periods in response to social forces.[31] Sometimes these identities are connected with particular subcultures (bohemians, hippies, goths, punks, bikers); occasionally, they are triggered by new medical techniques, such as the emergence of the identity of transsexual in the 1960s and '70s with the advent of new surgical techniques that made it possible to create and shape genitalia. What makes our contemporary neurobiological concepts different is the extent to which they have been promoted by pharmaceutical marketers. You are not shy; you have social anxiety disorder. You are not absentminded, dreamy, or fidgety; you have ADHD. You are not moody; you are bipolar. Each diagnosis comes with a prescription. Your need for medication becomes part of your identity.

•　　•　　•

Like many public relations specialists, Tom Nesi started off as a journalist. A native of New York City, Nesi attended Columbia University as an undergraduate and moved to the University of Southern California for graduate school in communications. When he finished USC, in 1973, Nesi began working as a freelance writer for any publication he could find— trade journals, the popular press, even television and movies. (He co-wrote an ABC movie called *Fight for Life* that starred Jerry Lewis, Morgan Freeman, and Patty Duke.) He became interested in medicine after helping a friend through an illness. "At the time, there really were no health journalists," Nesi says. "I would go to meetings and there would be two or three. It was not a big reporting beat." Nesi got many pitches from public relations people, who always seemed willing to buy him dinner. Some of these people became friends. When one of them put in a good word at the E. R. Squibb Corporation, a New Jersey–based pharmaceutical company, Nesi thought, *You know, I could get used to this life. Health benefits, a regular paycheck.* "I was thirty-four and it was time to settle down," he says.

Nesi spent the next twenty-five years in the pharmaceutical industry, first as public-affairs director for Squibb and later as a consultant to most of the other major companies through his own firm, TJN Communications. The Squibb complex was located just outside Princeton, where Nesi still lives. "It had a college feel to it, an academic feel," Nesi says. "There was a beautiful cafeteria overlooking the water." PR was not nearly as grand or as sinister as Bernays would have had us believe. Nesi spent a lot of time in marketing meetings. He wrote a lot of press releases. He set up interviews and cultivated relationships with physicians. "When you're in PR for a large corporation, you get really involved in corporate politics," Nesi says. "A lot of the things I did were about making friends, building alliances with people in Congress. I found myself doing for others what they had done for me. You'd go to meetings, talk to reporters, and take them out to dinner."

When Nesi began working at Squibb, in the early 1980s, the pharmaceutical industry looked much different than it does today. Most companies were led by men trained in science or medicine. The industry was solidly profitable, but not wildly so. It was slow to innovate, partly because patent law limited the availability of generic drugs. All this changed in the Reagan era. In 1984, the pharmaceutical market became much more competitive; the Hatch-Waxman Act made it easier and less expensive for generic-drug manufacturers to get their drugs approved. Venture capitalists began to invest in pharmaceuticals. Personal investment also started to take off, and pharmaceutical companies needed higher profit margins in order to attract investors. By the end of the decade, drug companies had begun to consolidate. Venerable companies with histories dating back to the nineteenth century, such as Upjohn, Searle, Burroughs Wellcome, Ciba, Sandoz, and Pharmacia, were either merged or taken over to form much larger, more powerful corporations, some of them with holdings that extended beyond pharmaceuticals to products such as food, perfume, and agriculture. In 1989, Squibb merged with the Bristol-Myers Company to form Bristol-Myers Squibb. Nesi says, "When Bristol-Myers bought the company, everything changed—everything. It just became one big bureaucracy."

For years, the pharmaceutical industry had resisted the idea of advertising drugs directly to consumers.[32] This was partly because advertising was considered rather vulgar but also because the companies had seen DTC advertising backfire. In the early 1980s Eli Lilly had marketed Oraflex, a nonsteroidal anti-inflammatory drug for arthritis, by sending out press kits not only to medical journals but also to mainstream media, including television and radio. By the standards of today, this tactic seems modest, but at the time it pushed the envelope of what was considered ethically acceptable. Oraflex got tremendous media coverage, and Lilly sold half a million prescriptions in the first fourteen weeks after it was launched. But Oraflex also proved toxic to the liver and kidneys, and it caused dozens of deaths in the United States and the United Kingdom before it was pulled from the market, in 1982.[33] For drug marketers concerned that DTC advertising would endanger patients, Oraflex was a cautionary tale. If you advertised drugs directly to consumers, you might actually harm more of them by encouraging them to take the drugs before the full spectrum of risks became apparent.

Of course, the industry also had a more mercenary reason for opposing DTC ads: it was much cheaper to market to physicians. Richard Hull, the marketing director for SmithKline and French, had made this point in a lecture to the National Pharmaceutical Council as early as 1958. To place a full-page ad in four medical journals cost about three thousand dollars, Hull said. To do the same thing in the four biggest popular magazines—*Life, Time,* the *Saturday Evening Post,* and *Reader's Digest*—cost eighty thousand dollars.[34] Why market to the masses when you could market to the gatekeepers? So in the early 1980s, when Congress considered a proposal to permit DTC ads, the major pharmaceutical companies were united in their opposition. The chief of Eli Lilly called it "unwise and inappropriate." The VP of American Home Products said that "DTC advertising would make [patients] extraordinarily susceptible to product promises." The chief of Bristol-Myers wrote, "We fail to understand a benefit to *any* audience."[35]

By the early 1990s, however, the atmosphere had begun to change. The new watchword was *patient empowerment.* In 1992 the AMA voted to reverse its opposition to DTC advertising. Two years later the American Association of Advertising Agencies teamed up with the Washington Legal Foundation, a libertarian pro-business group, to challenge the FDA's restrictions on DTC advertising. By this time many pharmaceutical companies were headed by businesspeople, rather than physicians, who were more than happy to advertise to consumers. In 1997, the FDA agreed to drop its brief-summary requirement, a misleadingly titled rule that required advertisements to consumers to include detailed (and not at all brief) descriptions of the side effects of drugs. These descriptions were often so long and complex that they made television advertising impossible. Once the brief-summary requirement was rolled back, however, the gates were wide open for drug ads on TV.

"It has been a disaster for the industry, a complete disaster," Nesi says. "It's almost as if you can trace the decline of the stocks in the pharmaceutical industry with the rise of DTC advertising." For years pharmaceutical companies had been marketing their drugs solely to doctors, and they had developed a reliable strategy: you detail doctors in their offices, you give them lunch and drug samples, and you place ads in their journals. Suddenly the companies found themselves in the strange new world of Madison Avenue, where the customs were unfamiliar, the natives were treacherous, and the bills were shockingly high. "Pharmaceutical companies had no experience dealing with Madison Avenue, I mean none," Nesi says. "And then all of a sudden they are being confronted with: well, you've got to spend a hundred million here, a couple hundred million there. These guys had no background in that. This was not the pharmaceutical business."

Consumer marketing made for a jarring contrast with the old days. Back in the 1980s, Nesi says, "I once heard my boss dress down a product manager for spending twenty-five thousand dollars. He had taken out a series of four-page color spreads in the *New England Journal of Medicine.* Twenty-five thousand dollars!" Once the restrictions on television advertising were lifted, however, the financial stakes shot up dramatically. Launching a drug was like playing in a high-rolling poker game where you had to flash a fat bankroll just to get a seat at the table. "Before DTC advertising, a huge amount of money to spend on marketing expenses for the launch of a drug could be measured in the tens of millions. Now it's hundreds of millions," Nesi says. "To launch Vioxx alone, for the television advertising you're talking about two hundred and fifty million. Well, when you're talking about that kind of money to launch a product, you have to generate the profit and the sales to support that money. You don't have the luxury of rolling a drug out slowly and seeing what's going to happen. You have to hit the market with a bang."

From a purely business perspective, DTC advertising worked like a charm. The worries about expenses that Richard Hull expressed in 1958 —why sell to the masses when for much less money you can target the people holding the prescription pads?—proved misguided. According to a 2003 study by the Kaiser Family Foundation, each dollar spent on DTC advertising yielded an additional $4.20 in sales. This return on investment was far greater than that of advertising aimed at physicians.[36] By 2005, eight years after the FDA relaxed its ban, drug marketers had seen the dividends of DTC ads pay off. Spending on DTC advertising had increased by 330 percent, to a total of $29.9 billion annually.[37]

As Lilly discovered with its disastrous Oraflex experiment, however, DTC marketing also came with serious hazards. Exhibit number one was, yet again, Vioxx, the notorious pain drug that Merck was forced to withdraw from the market in 2004 (and which, as we have seen in earlier chapters, was promoted with ghostwritten articles, phony medical journals, and intimidation of academic critics). Not only was Vioxx the top-selling drug for Merck at the time it was pulled from the market, generating $20 billion in sales, it was also one of the most heavily advertised drugs in America. When Vioxx was withdrawn, many industry observers were stunned—including Nesi, who had consulted for Merck. "My initial reaction was it was some kind of freakish event," Nesi said in an interview with journalist Ed Silverman. "I didn't think there could have been much behind it. I've seen things like that before happen in clinical trials—side effects show up and drugs get taken off the market. Anybody who's worked in a pharma company has seen failures in trials and knows it is part of the business. But to see a failure after $20 billion in sales is really quite extraordinary."[38]

Nesi began looking into the Vioxx story with the aim of defending the pharmaceutical industry. He felt sure that Merck was getting a bad rap. But the deeper he dug into the case, the more alarmed he became. Soon he was staying up until 3:00 a.m. reading Merck memos. What shocked him was the sheer breadth of the deception and intimidation Merck had used to promote Vioxx—an effort that involved billions of marketing dollars and implicated the FDA, academic thought leaders, medical ghostwriters, and the *New England Journal of Medicine*. "I was absolutely furious at what Merck had done," Nesi says. "Everybody would say, How could you have done something like that? I didn't do that! I would never do that! Never in a million years would my corporation or I have put out those press releases, or said things, or done things like that." Nesi was especially dismayed by the actions of the public relations office. "PR people used to consider themselves the conscience of the corporation, and lots of the battles I used to have at Squibb were with the marketing people," Nesi says. At Merck, however, the public relations people were part of the deception. "Instead of stopping it, they basically helped." In 2008, Nesi published a scathingly critical book about the Vioxx scandal called *Poison Pills.*

As Nesi points out, Vioxx was no ordinary drug withdrawal. For one thing, it affected an extraordinary number of patients. At the time Vioxx was taken off the market, it was being prescribed to roughly two million people, many of whom took it regularly for chronic pain. When the bulk of the lawsuits against Merck were settled four years later, the bill came to $4.85 billion, one of the largest civil settlements in history.[39] (However, that settlement was still dwarfed by the massive $21.1 billion Wyeth has set aside to settle the Fen-Phen litigation.) [40] Another reason the Vioxx scandal stood out was simply that it implicated Merck, which had carefully cultivated an image as the most buttoned-down, socially responsible, research-driven member of the pharmaceutical club. Yet the more information that emerged, the more spectacularly crooked Merck appeared to be—intentionally misrepresenting research results, distributing ghostwritten articles, paying a publisher to develop fake medical journals, even sending out a corporate vice president to intimidate the drug's critics. Long after the dangers of Vioxx were clear to many outside experts, Merck was still doing its best to make the drug appear safe.

In the immediate aftermath of the Vioxx scandal, many industry critics pointed to DTC advertising as the culprit. Television ads had allowed Merck to launch Vioxx quickly and push it furiously, before its dangers became fully evident. There was a brief backlash. "I do think that one of things we are going to learn is that direct-to-consumer advertising created a monster here," said the Cleveland Clinic's Dr. Eric Topol, a prominent Vioxx critic, in 2004.[41] Yet it was not long before consumers lost their fear of the monster. While Merck eventually settled a multistate lawsuit over its Vioxx advertising, paying out $58 million to twenty-nine states and the District of Columbia for allegedly deceptive advertising, DTC advertising actually increased in the years following the scandal. [42] Not until the financial downturn of 2008 was it finally scaled back.

In fact, DTC advertising was only one piece of a deeper problem, which was the blockbuster-drug model. The blockbuster model encouraged companies to work on drugs for mild, chronic conditions that affected a large number of people, then market the drugs as frenetically as possible before the patents expired. DTC advertising simply took the pressures of the blockbuster model and ramped up their intensity. In 1992, there were only four blockbuster drugs on the market. According to IMS Health, by 2006, nine years after the restrictions on DTC advertising were lifted, the number of blockbusters had leaped to ninety-two.[43] Once a company has so much money riding on the success of a single drug, it faces enormous pressure to have that drug succeed; if it fails, the entire future of the company might be jeopardized. As Tom Nesi points out, a single Pfizer drug—the cholesterol-lowering drug Lipitor—is now worth more than the entire company of Squibb was worth when Bristol-Myers bought it in 1990. This kind of financial pressure can lead people to actions that would otherwise have been unthinkable. "Talking to my friends now, who still work in pharma, they hate it," Nesi says. "The old-fashioned drug reps used to go out and play golf with the doctors on Wednesday. Now it's mass marketing."

•　•　•

Of all the PR innovations credited to Bernays, perhaps the simplest and most durable has been a tactic known as the third-party technique. As the name suggests, this strategy simply means getting your message into the mouth of a disinterested third party, preferably a recognized expert. In his 1928 book *Propaganda,* Bernays gave the example of a meatpacker client who wanted to sell bacon. An ordinary advertiser would simply counsel the meatpacker to devise an ad explaining that bacon is inexpensive, that it is good for you, that it gives you energy, or any number of other positive things about bacon, most of which will not make people buy bacon. The public relations counsel asks a very different question. He wants to know: "Who is it that influences the eating habits of the public?" The answer, Bernays wrote, is physicians. Bernays recruited five thousand physicians to endorse a hearty meal of bacon and eggs for breakfast and then publicized the "survey" to the newspapers, where it was reported as news. The result, he claimed, was a satisfying increase in bacon sales.[44] "If you can influence the leaders, either with or without their conscious cooperation," Bernays wrote, "you automatically influence the group which they sway."

To a modern consumer, the bacon survey that Bernays devised sounds quaint and gimmicky, like those 1950s magazine ads that featured smiling doctors telling people what brand of cigarettes was the healthiest. This is partly because marketing styles have changed, but it is also because our sources of authority have shifted. Today, you cannot simply take a survey of doctors; you need a randomized, controlled trial, conducted out of a major research center, published in a reputable journal, and publicized by a university communications office. Even so, the fundamental principle behind the third-party technique has endured. A message carries more impact if it comes from a source that is credible and unbiased.

For years, the most credible authorities were physicians. That has changed, however, according to Lydia Worthington. The new authorities are just as likely to be patients. Worthington is a vice president with BuzzMetrics, a division of Nielsen, Inc., that specializes in tracking online consumer buzz. Pharmaceuticals are their largest area of growth. Worthington says that pharma companies now target opinion leaders among patient support groups in the same way that they target physicians. "In specific depression groups, there are patients who have almost as much knowledge, or more knowledge, than a medical professional, just because they are involved in this personally. And they've done all the research, and know everything that's going on, and they are giving specific drug advice out," Worthington says. "From our point of view, and now also from the pharmaceutical industry point of view, they are as important as your physician opinion leaders." Worthington advises companies to reach out to patients who are especially influential online, such as bloggers and Twitterers. "You treat them almost the same way you'd treat a medical journalist," she says. "They are your press."

The emergence of patients as a serious social force began in the Reagan era, when a generation of baby boomers began to enter middle age. Nurtured on the consumer rights movement of the 1960s and '70s, these patients were unwilling to sit back passively while physicians and bureaucrats made their medical decisions. They wanted a voice of their own. Many organized themselves into formal advocacy groups. The most visible of these groups were AIDS activists, such as ACT UP. Faced with a lethal epidemic and no real treatment in sight, activists began demanding more research on AIDS and greater access to clinical trials. The AIDS activists were unlike any patient groups that had come before. They were not quiet, behind-the-scenes operators. They backed their demands with guerrilla tactics closer to those of the anti-war protesters of the 1960s. "I remember they chained themselves in the New York Stock Exchange," says Tom Nesi. "Trading stopped on our stock." As pharmaceutical companies were forced to take the demands of AIDS activists seriously, other advocacy groups took notice and asked, "What about us?"

An answer came from the Pharmaceutical Manufacturers Association (PMA). In 1985 Gerry Mossinghoff, a former official in the patent and trademark office of the Reagan administration, became head of the PMA. As Greg Critser points out in his book *Generation Rx*, Mossinghoff saw the rising power of patients as a prime political opportunity. He put together an organization called the Healthcare Quality Alliance (HQA), which the PMA underwrote and housed in its headquarters. The mission of the HQA was to coordinate and support patient organizations, such as the American Diabetes Association and the American Cancer Society. At first the HQA just lobbied for more basic research funding at the NIH. But soon they moved on to more ambitious goals. Mossinghoff encouraged companies to invite patient advocacy groups to their plants in order to build trust. If a company was anticipating trouble getting a new drug approved, it could brief the group in advance about how to testify at an FDA advisory-board meeting. If Medicare stopped paying for an expensive drug, the HQA would send a brigade of patients to visit the Hill and educate Congress about the consequences. Joe Isaacs, who worked with the PMA, told Critser, "We basically created a disease-of-the-month club."[45]

The strategy paid off. Merck, for instance, devised a plan to work with AIDS activists by setting up a corporate advisory committee. According to John Doorley, the head of corporate communications at Merck in the early 1990s, the company realized it could not work with every AIDS activist. "So we tried reaching out to a few and have them work as ambassadors," Doorley said. Later, when San Francisco activists planned to protest against Merck, they were stopped by the committee. Doorley said, "They called the guys in San Francisco and said, 'You go to any other company you want to, but not Merck.'"[46]

In some ways, the alliance between pharma companies and patients made perfect sense. The companies saw patients as ideal third-party advocates for their drugs: unbiased sources whose authority came from personal experience. Patient advocacy groups, in turn, saw drug research as their best hope for fighting illness, so they pressed an agenda that lined up favorably with that of industry: more clinical trials, faster drug approvals, and more funding for research. Advocacy groups were also usually strapped for money, and they depended on charitable contributions for their survival. If pharmaceutical companies could fill the gap, most groups were happy to take advantage of their generosity. Today virtually every patient advocacy group in the country relies on industry support. The Depression and Bipolar Support Alliance gets over half its funding from industry. For the Colorectal Cancer Coalition, the figure is 81 percent.[47] Over the past several years the National Alliance for Mental Illness (NAMI) has received two thirds of its donations from industry.[48] For a time, NAMI was even led by an executive on loan from Eli Lilly.[49]

Advocacy groups argue that simply taking money from industry does not mean complicity in industry aims. But sometimes the charge of complicity is hard to refute. In the early 1990s, a patient group called the Human Growth Foundation began sponsoring a screening program in the public schools of Atlanta, Georgia. One aim of the Human Growth Foundation was to raise awareness of growth disorders, such as human growth hormone deficiency. To that end, the foundation began train gym teachers in the Atlanta public schools to measure the growth of school-children with specialized equipment and plot the growth on a chart. If a child ranked in the bottom fifth percentile, the school sent a letter to the parents of the child, urging them to contact their physicians or the Human Growth Foundation.

To critics, however, these growth measurements were not simply about children's health. The largest financial backer of the Human Growth Foundation at the time was Genentech, the San Francisco–based biotechnology company. And there was a good reason why Genentech was so eager to support the group: Genentech manufactures a synthetic version of human growth hormone, which is used mainly to treat children with short stature. At the time of the screening program, the growth hormone cost between twenty thousand and forty thousand dollars a year; children were often treated for as long as ten years.[50] Although human growth hormone was initially approved by the FDA to treat children who were short because of growth hormone deficiency, its use was gradually expanded to include children who were short for other medical reasons, such as chronic kidney disease or Turner's syndrome. Some pediatricians were also prescribing growth hormone for children who were simply short, even though there was little evidence that the hormone would significantly increase the child's stature as an adult.

The industry donations to the program were not inconsiderable. The Atlanta screening program was funded by a hundred-thousand-dollar donation from Genentech, which controlled 70 percent of the growth hormone market. The other 30 percent of the market was controlled by Eli Lilly, which was the second-largest donor to the Human Growth Foundation. Both Genentech and Lilly had executives representing them on the foundation's advisory board. Critics were naturally suspicious that the screening tests were merely a tool to expand the market for growth hormone, but the executive director of the foundation dismissed these suspicions. The tests were just a warning signal for parents, she told the *Wall Street Journal*, adding: "They are not a veiled marketing attempt."[51]

It is no coincidence that the rising power of patients as drug marketers came at a time when the authority and prestige of physicians was declining. As physicians began to see themselves more and more as businesspeople in the 1980s and 1990s, their independent authority as professionals waned. If physicians are trying to sell you something, you can no longer assume they have your best interests at heart. Patients, on the other hand, are in a different position. At least on the surface, patients do not have any obvious financial interest in marketing a drug. Nor do they have deep medical knowledge. Their authority comes from another place—not scientific training or clinical expertise, but firsthand experience of an illness and its treatment. In public relations, their role is to front a marketing campaign and give it a sympathetic human face.

In 2001, for instance, the pharmaceutical companies Pfizer and Eisai were promoting Aricept, a drug intended to slow the progression of Alzheimer's disease. Because Alzheimer's is diagnosed solely by the patient's symptoms (no diagnostic laboratory or imaging tests are available), the disorder was a promising candidate for a disease-awareness campaign. So in concert with the Alzheimer's Association, a Chicago-based patient group, Pfizer and Eisai hired two public relations companies to publicize the disease: Hill and Knowlton, the international PR giant, and TBWA Health, a smaller company specializing in health-care communications. To drive home the message that Alzheimer's was unfairly stigmatized, this public relations team orchestrated a remarkably effective series of media events. First they produced a public-service announcement with the Alzheimer's Association that featured clips of Rita Hayworth, a victim of Alzheimer's who died in 1987. Then they recruited Hayworth's daughter to unveil the PSA at the World Alzheimer's Congress. Finally, in a publicity tactic worthy of a postmodern cultural theorist, they filmed VNRs of the unveiling of their own PSA—thus generating both the fake news event and the fake news coverage of the event. The public relations team even persuaded a producer of the television show *ER* to write Aricept into an episode that starred Alan Alda as a doctor with early-stage Alzheimer's.

The campaign returned impressive results. Several hundred reporters came to the Alzheimer's congress, many of them from international news organizations. The Rita Hayworth PSA ran 12,000 times on 257 stations. President Clinton announced a $50 million NIH funding package for research on Alzheimer's disease, and *Time* magazine ran a cover story. In only ten days, the campaign recorded over eight hundred million media impressions—more than the Alzheimer's Association usually gets in an entire year. So effective was the public relations campaign that it was awarded two Recognizing Excellence awards for "raising awareness about a previously disregarded disease."[52]

Over time, such disease-awareness campaigns have settled into a familiar pattern. A pharmaceutical company funds studies showing that an illness is undertreated. A medical communications company recruits a team of thought leaders to lend their academic authority to the campaign. A public relations firm engineers an event to promote awareness of the disease, such as National Bladder Health Week or Walk for a Cure. Finally, a patient advocacy group provides compelling stories of human suffering, preferably with a celebrity patient on the talk show circuit. Lauren Hutton was one of the first such celebrity patients; she appeared in *Parade* magazine in 2000.[53] Her talking points were about hormone replacement therapy; her check came from Wyeth. Hutton proved so appealing that other celebrities lined up to follow suit. NFL running back Ricky Williams chatted to interviewers about his debilitating social anxiety disorder; he was funded by GlaxoSmithKline, the maker of Paxil. Cybill Shepherd talked about irritable bowel syndrome courtesy of Novartis, the maker of Zelnorm. Bob Dole discussed erectile dysfunction on behalf of Pfizer, the maker of Viagra. Today celebrity patients are so successful that speakers' bureaus will even pair celebrity patients with companies that need disease spokespeople.[54]

Not all of these arrangements work out well, of course. In 2004 Bristol-Myers Squibb recruited Andy Behrman, the author of *Electroboy*, a memoir of bipolar disorder, to be a spokesperson for its antipsychotic drug Abilify. Behrman was an unlikely spokesman. According to his memoir, he had served five months in prison for art forgery, cheated his friends and family out of thousands of dollars for a failed film project, and even worked for a time as a male stripper. His diagnosis was bipolar disorder, a condition for which Abilify had not even been approved. Yet over the next four years Bristol-Myers Squibb paid Behrman more than four hundred thousand dollars. In return, Behrman spoke from the script provided by the PR agency, emphasizing that the drug had saved him from his illness and its other treatments. "Since I switched to Abilify, almost all the side effects have gone away," he said in a promotional video.

Three years later, however, Behrman recanted everything, telling the press that he had actually felt worse on Abilify than on any other drug he had ever tried. According to BMS, the relationship with Behrman turned sour when Behrman demanded $7.5 million to keep speaking positively about their drug.[55]

Probably the most ill-conceived third-party tactic of recent years came several years ago from PhRMA, the pharmaceutical trade group. Because American drug prices are so high (the highest in the world, by far), many Americans have begun buying their drugs from Canada, where a drug may cost as little as a tenth of what it does in the United States. This cross-border buying was making a serious dent in drug industry profits. To discourage the practice, PhRMA commissioned a ghostwriter, Julie Chrystyn, to produce a thriller about Croatian Muslim terrorists who attack Americans by poisoning drugs sold through Canadian pharmacies. The ghostwriter called it *The Spivak Conspiracy,* named for a friend of hers, Kenin Spivak, who later joined her in writing the book. (The proposed editor of the novel was Jayson Blair, the notorious *New York Times* writer who was dismissed for fabricating and plagiarizing news stories.)

Although the writers produced their thriller in less than two months, the deal eventually fell apart. Mark Barondess, the PhRMA consultant who brokered the agreement, rejected the manuscript on the grounds that it was poorly written. (On the NPR show *On the Media,* he claimed that it was so bad that readers would need Dramamine to get past the third chapter.)[56] He offered the writers $100,000 to keep quiet. The writers rejected the money and rewrote the book, eventually publishing it under the title *The Karasik Conspiracy.* In the new version, the villain is no longer a Croatian terrorist organization. It is a multinational pharmaceutical company that selectively poisons drugs sold in Canada in an effort to frighten Americans away from buying drugs abroad.[57]

•　•　•

"I was in the exam room waiting for my doctor," says Joel Roselin, beginning to describe the moment of his epiphany. Joel had spent nearly his entire lifetime working in pharmaceutical marketing. As he looked around, he saw an examining room filled with industry knickknacks and brochures. Immediately he thought of his doctor: "I hope he's getting his information from the medical literature and not from people like me." If there was any single incident that drove Joel out of pharmaceutical marketing, it was that one. "That's when I realized that I was part of a big scam," he says. "Either the stuff I was putting out was not having an impact, which meant that lots of people were making lots of money and driving up the cost of drugs for nothing, or the stuff was affecting prescribing behavior and undermining my own care." Soon after, Joel left marketing and enrolled in Harvard Divinity School.

Joel and I have known each other for years, mainly from the bioethics conference circuit. He has freckles and reddish hair, and his default facial expression seems to be a wry, easygoing grin. When we first met he was working at Harvard Medical School, coordinating the ethics teaching program for medical students. Now he works in research ethics at Columbia University. Joel is also one of the few people in America who marketed drugs as a child. His father owned a television production company in New York that produced VNRs, mainly for the pharmaceutical industry. Joel appeared in his first VNR when he was five or six years old. "That's why my dad had kids, because talent was too expensive," he says. Joel worked summers in the mail room, and when he finished college, he started working full-time in the family business. Later he moved to Burson-Marsteller, an international public relations firm, and then to a major advertising company. "My first account at Burson-Marsteller was for an over-the-counter product called Equalactin," he says. Equalactin is a drug for bowel complaints. Joel says, "The brilliant ad campaign was the 'tortoise and the hare.'" Here he puts on a mocking, adman voice: "Because sometimes you go too fast, and sometimes you go too slow."

In the world of medicine, there seem to be two broad categories of people who see the drug industry as a problem. One group sees the issue in formal, bureaucratic terms. They take the same matter-of-fact attitude toward excessive influence as they do toward traffic violations or restaurants that cut corners with the health code. For a handful of people, however, the discomfort with industry influence seems more visceral. Their necks prickle when they hear patients called "customers" or a hospital unit referred to as a "revenue generator." Joel seems to fall into this latter group. He enjoyed the intellectual challenge of public relations, but the salesmanship made him want to reach for the Equalactin. "I didn't like going out to dinner with clients," he says. "I felt smarmy."

Yet it is not a stretch to imagine him as a salesman. He is warm and funny, a natural performer with a sharp intellect who counters his extroversion with subtle self-mockery. But he is also self-aware enough to understand that these traits could be effectively deployed as selling tools, which is precisely what made him queasy. "I felt like I was trading on something that was very personal, which was my personality," Joel says. In the ad business, he explains, there are discrete areas: copywriters, art directors, and account people. "I was an account person," he says. "So what does that mean? I don't write copy, I don't do artistic work, so what do I do? I keep the client happy. Talk about feeling like a whore!"

When Joel was selling VNRs for his father's company in the 1980s, he was once asked to entertain the young protégé of one of their valued pharmaceutical clients. "He was your classic pharma guy," says Joel. "He had been an athlete, a really handsome, all-American type guy." At one point in the evening, the guy turned to Joel and said, "Do you know any good strip clubs?" (Joel adds that this question came just after the guy told him about his wife and children.) Strip clubs were one topic about which Joel had no knowledge or interest. The only clubs he could think of were the seedy, low-end places in Times Square, next to the quarter peep shows. "It was gross," he says. "They served you beer in cans, and I had to sit there next to this guy and make small talk, and that just grossed me out. I thought, *Is this what you have to do in this business? I'd rather be up there with the girls dancing with my clothes off than sitting here with this schlemiel.*"

Although Joel participated in his share of flackery over the years, he took a skeptical attitude toward the more outrageous PR stunts. He never joined in unlikely schemes such as PhRMA's ghosted Croatian thriller. "The problems occur when someone gets a dumb idea and there are no lawyers around to tell them not to do it," Joel says. Advertising and PR people all think their ideas are brilliant. "And they think they're smarter than everyone else, kind of like criminals who think they've figured out the perfect crime. But if no one has done it before, there's probably a really good reason." Once, Joel had a boss who was trying to figure out a way to make sure that men in minority communities took their ACE inhibitors, a category of blood pressure drugs. "He jokingly suggested putting the drug in a condom, like a transdermal patch, and calling it 'ACE in the hole.' Who knows if some idiot marketer might not have thought that was a good idea."

It may have been inevitable that Joel would leave the business. In order to be a really good marketer, he says, you need to really believe in what you are selling. A sincere evangelist will save more souls than one plagued by self-doubt. But Joel could never quite convince himself that he was working for a righteous cause, and now he wonders whether his doubts made his colleagues uncomfortable. Perhaps the presence of a heretic undermined the confidence of everyone else. "There is definitely a kind of contamination of the unbeliever," he says. "They have to be cast out."

Even before Joel had his epiphany in the examining room, he was growing uneasy about the ethics of his job. It is not that drug marketers have no sense of morality, he points out. "They can engage with you in a moral debate about what they do," he says. "But they can only do it through the lens of financial success." When Joel worked in medical advertising, he used to schmooze with one of his bosses over coffee. The two of them got along well, and Joel felt comfortable joking around with him. One day Joel asked, "If someone asked you to promote a product you thought was dangerous, would you do it?" His boss paused and thought about the question for a while. Eventually he came up with an answer: "I'd like to think we wouldn't."

CHAPTER SIX

The Ethicists

EVERAL YEARS AGO, local television news stations began running news segments about Xigris, a sepsis drug produced by Eli Lilly. Sepsis is an infection of the blood that can threaten the lives of hospital patients. "Robert Lieberman is lucky to be alive," reported a New York station. "He was on a ventilator near death when he got a new biotech drug called Xigris that probably saved his life." The reporter noted that while Xigris had been a lifesaver, it was also very expensive, raising troubling ethical questions. Should patients be denied the drug because of its expense?

When Lilly launched Xigris, in 2001, it hoped that the drug would be a blockbuster. Prozac, another Lilly drug, had recently lost its patent protection, and the company needed a replacement. But Xigris had not taken off. One reason may have been that Xigris was no better than older treatments for sepsis. The main reason, however, was its cost. Standard treatments for sepsis usually cost less than $50 per day, while Xigris cost $6,800 per treatment. So Lilly hired a public relations agency called Belsito and Company to promote the drug. Belsito designed a public relations campaign called the Ethics, the Urgency, and the Potential, and its premise was that it is "unethical *not* to use the drug." To reinforce the point, Lilly funded a $1.8 million project called the Values, Ethics, and Rationing in Critical Care (VERICC) Task Force, in which bioethicists and physicians from various American medical schools examined the ethics of rationing certain drugs and services.[1] It was VERICC that made the evening news.

The strategy was brilliant. There is no better way to enlist bioethicists in the cause of consumer capitalism than to convince them they are working for social justice. Many bioethicists see it as part of their job description to write and speak on behalf of those who are ill, disadvantaged, or oppressed. In the words of one prominent practitioner, bioethics is intimately concerned "with liberty, with rights struggle, and with the drama of the one against the powerful authorities."[2] Apparently, bioethicists are also a good vehicle for selling drugs. When the PR campaign was finished, the Council on Public Relations highlighted the VERICC Task Force as a successful case study, pointing out that VERICC drew 60 media outlets, attracted more than 132 million viewers, and was covered by the *Wall Street Journal,* National Public Radio, ABC *World News Tonight,* the *Toronto Star,* and the *Boston Globe.* By early 2004, Xigris sales were up 36 percent.[3]

Given the dismal reputation of the pharmaceutical industry, you might think that ethicists would be reluctant to join forces with it. Yet in the late 1990s, it became clear that industry was funding bioethics in a variety of different ways. Many ethicists did not see this as a problem. It's not like a doctor taking industry money, they argued; ethicists generally don't write prescriptions. And it's not really like a regulator taking money either. Bioethicists don't control drug approval or issue black-box warnings. In the eyes of many bioethicists, it's more like funding a charity. Drug industry executives have so much money they can barely keep it from spilling out of their pockets. Bioethicists make the world a better place. Why shouldn't they be paid?

The argument is not that far-fetched. Unlike some academic fields, bioethics has a strong undercurrent of social activism. Many ethicists would like to think their job is not merely to study the world but to change it. And as any community organizer, human rights worker, or environmental activist can tell you, changing the world costs money. Many charitable organizations have been built out of the fortunes of ruthlessly driven American businessmen. To many ethicists, accepting money from the pharmaceutical industry does not mean endorsing its marketing practices, any more than accepting money from the federal government means endorsing its foreign policy. You take the money and use it for a good cause.

In fact, bioethics has become a cause in itself. For the past three decades bioethics has been vigorously generating new centers, new commissions, new journals, and new graduate programs, not to mention a highly politicized role in American public life. In the same way that sociologists saw their fortunes climb during the 1960s as the public eye turned toward social issues like poverty, crime, and education, bioethics started to ascend when medical care and scientific research began generating social questions of their own. As the field grows more prominent, bioethicists are considering a funding model familiar to the realm of business ethics, one that embraces partnership and collaboration with corporate sponsors as long as outright conflicts of interest can be managed. This funding model allows, for example, the nonprofit Ethics Resource Center in Washington, D.C., to sponsor ethics and leadership programs funded by the tobacco industry and weapons manufacturers.[4] Similarly, Harold Shapiro, a former president of Princeton University, drew an annual director's salary from Dow Chemical Company while serving as chair of the National Bioethics Advisory Commission during the Clinton administration. Meanwhile, Dow had famously been the defendant in a highly publicized lawsuit over the Dow Corning silicone breast implants, as well as in numerous legal actions involving disposal of hazardous waste.[5]

Corporate funding presents a public relations challenge, of course. It looks unseemly for an ethicist to share in the profits of arms dealers, industrial polluters, or multinationals that exploit the developing world. Credibility is also a concern. Bioethicists teach about pharmaceutical company issues in university classrooms, write about those issues in books and articles, and comment on them in the press. Many bioethicists evaluate industry policies and practices for professional boards, government bodies, and research ethics committees. To critics, this raises legitimate questions about the field of bioethics itself. Where does the authority of ethicists come from, and why are corporations so willing to fund them?

•   •   •

A few years ago, I got an e-mail from the CEO of a now-defunct company called Foreview inviting me to become part of its "global network of experts." Foreview was sort of a corporate-academic dating service. It matched up academic experts with businesses seeking expertise. According to its Web site, Foreview provided its clients with "information about tomorrow's state of the economy and politics." It did this partly through its Ask the Experts service, which hired people like me to respond to questions posed by clients. My payment for taking part in Ask the Experts would be $175 per question. I was also told that this work would probably lead to more detailed consulting projects for which I could set my own rates, although Foreview would receive a 10 percent finder's fee, capped at a maximum of $5,000.

I did not take Foreview up on its offer, which sounded a little too much like a Dear Abby column, but I did start to ask colleagues in bioethics about the kinds of corporate consultations they had been asked to do. The type of work available varies: testifying as an expert witness in court cases, preparing reports, giving talks at industry-sponsored meetings (often held at ski resorts or foreign vacation spots). A handful of pharmaceutical companies have hired their own in-house ethicists, but most seem to rely on consultants from the academic world. Evan DeRenzo, a staff member at the Center for Ethics at Washington Hospital Center, told me she charges Janssen Pharmaceuticals by the hour to sit in on meetings, review research protocols, and help the company develop policy and educational sessions.

Bioethics has always had an ambivalent relationship with power. The field emerged in the 1960s, when protesting against authority was practically a generational requirement for those of a certain age, and many ethicists see it as their role to speak for the powerless—for patients against doctors, for research subjects against sponsors, for the medically underserved against the insurers and the bureaucrats. Like any new field, bioethics has struggled to establish its legitimacy; bioethicists must be taken seriously if their work is going to have any effect. As the field has come of age, however, many bioethicists have grown uneasy with their rising status. It is one thing to be a social critic and another thing entirely to be the voice of moral authority. Some scholars have recoiled, emphatically rejecting the notion that their voices should count more than others' on ethical affairs. A few cringe at the term *bioethicist,* which carries a slightly self-important air of professionalism and expertise. Yet others display their moral authority like a newly promoted captain showing off his stripes. For them, bioethics is a professional service that deserves social respect, market compensation, and the occasional appearance on a television news program.

A handful of bioethicists have started their own businesses. When Glenn McGee was unexpectedly dismissed as director of the Alden March Bioethics Center at Albany Medical School, he registered a for-profit consulting business called BENE, or the Bioethics Education Network, LLC. He told the *Business Review* that he was "trying to build what will become at least a $500,000 business in Albany."[6] David Perlman used to work as an ethicist for GlaxoSmithKline; today he works at the University of Pennsylvania, where he has founded Eclipse Ethics Education Enterprises, LLC. (He is also identified as "the inventor of the Crucial Choices learning format," which is based on his experience at GlaxoSmithKline developing "ethics cases wrapped around a Jeopardy-type game format for our senior leadership teams."[7]) Bruce Weinstein, who markets himself as the "Ethics Guy," was a faculty member in bioethics at the West Virginia University Health Sciences Center before he started a for-profit service called Ethics at Work. He has published a series of self-help ethics books offering moral advice on everything from dating to personal hygiene. You can measure your "ethics IQ" on his Web site.[8]

Other scholars have entered the consultation market in a more modest way. In the late 1990s, when issues such as human cloning and embryonic stem cell research first became topics of heated ethical discussion, many biotechnology companies began setting up bioethics advisory boards. These boards meet periodically to consider issues and offer the companies advice. A list of those reported to have served on such advisory boards reads like a who's who of bioethics: Nancy Dubler of Montefiore Medical for DNA Sciences; Ronald Green of Dartmouth for Advanced Cell Technology; Arthur Caplan of the University of Pennsylvania for Celera Genomics and DuPont; Karen Lebacqz of the Pacific School of Religion and Laurie Zoloth of Northwestern for Geron Corporation.[9] Consultation fees vary considerably. According to the *New York Times*, in 2001 Advanced Cell Technology was paying its advisory-board members a mere two hundred dollars per meeting while Geron paid a thousand dollars. Celera compensated Arthur Caplan annually in stock options; he converted them to cash and donated the money to the Center for Bioethics at the University of Pennsylvania, which he directs. One year that stock was worth more than a hundred thousand dollars.

Not surprisingly, these industry payments began to generate ethical questions of their own. Barbara Koenig, then at Stanford University, said that she was paid two thousand dollars per meeting for one corporate ethics board, an amount that troubled her. "I realized that the only reason I was going to this was because I was getting paid," she said. "And that raised a red flag, and I immediately resigned."[10] But many bioethicists insist that they are learning from their industry relationships and shaping company policy for the better. Over the years, the list of bioethics advisers to industry has grown: Jonathan Moreno of the University of Pennsylvania for GlaxoSmithKline, James Childress of Virginia for Johnson and Johnson, Tom Beauchamp of Georgetown and Robert Levine of Yale for Eli Lilly.[11] A task force commissioned by the two major American professional bioethics bodies, the American Society for Bioethics and Humanities and the American Society of Law, Medicine and Ethics, concluded that private corporations should be encouraged to seek out paid bioethics consultants, because "bioethics will have an impact on that [corporate] activity only if bioethicists can be part of the dialogue." In fact, the task force did not merely encourage bioethics consultation; it suggested that bioethicists might consider advertising their services. (Interestingly, the task force refused to disclose the names of the companies for which its members had consulted.)[12]

Defenders of corporate consultation often bristle at the suggestion that accepting money from industry compromises their impartiality or makes them any less objective as moral critics. "Objectivity is a myth," DeRenzo told me, marshaling arguments from feminist philosophy to bolster her cause. "I don't think there is a person alive who is engaged in an activity who has absolutely no interest in how it will turn out." Thomas Donaldson, director of the ethics program at the Wharton School, has compared ethics consultants to the external accounting firms often employed by corporations to audit their financial records.[13] Like accountants, ethicists may be paid by the very industries they are assessing, but they are kept honest by the need to maintain a reputation for integrity.

But ethical analysis does not really resemble a financial audit. If a company is cooking its books and the accountant closes his eyes to this fact in his audit, the accountant's wrongdoing can be reliably detected and verified by outside monitors. It is not so easy with an ethics consultant. Ethicists have widely divergent views. They come from different religious standpoints, use different theoretical frameworks, and profess different political philosophies. They are also free to change their minds at any point. How do you tell the difference between an ethics consultant who has changed her mind for legitimate reasons and one who has changed her mind for money? What distinguishes the consultant who has been hired for her integrity from the one who has been hired because her moral viewpoint lines up nicely with that of company executives?

In *Merchants of Immortality,* a book that examines the history of the biotechnology industry, Stephen Hall offers little evidence that the teams of bioethicists contracted by two biotechnology companies, Geron and Advanced Cell Technology, played any meaningful role in shaping company policy. In one case, Hall calls the ethical review a "midwife to fundraising." His assessment is reinforced by Michael West, the biologist-entrepreneur who founded Geron and who later became CEO of Advanced Cell Technology. When questioned about the ethicists he recruited to advise Advanced Cell Technology on their ethically controversial research, West answered, "In the field of ethics, there are no ground rules, so it's just one ethicist's opinion versus another ethicist's opinion.

. . . You're not getting whether something is right or wrong, because it all depends on who you pick."[14] Few executives will pick an ethicist who wants to put the brakes on the corporate mission.

West's comment highlights a problem with ethics consultation. Any ethical problem can be approached from many different perspectives, each of which will come with its own subtleties and nuances and compromises. It is entirely possible that puzzled executives may want to hire an ethicist to guide them through some perilous terrain. However, they might also simply want a congenial, like-minded ethicist to provide cover for what they plan to do anyway. And to the ethicist who is hired, this will not feel like a moral compromise. It will feel like working with an ally.

Consider the case of Eli Lilly, which found itself in the media spotlight in 1996 when the *Wall Street Journal* reported that for two decades the company had been paying homeless alcoholics to test drugs at its Phase I clinic in Indianapolis.[15] Company officials insisted that the homeless subjects were driven by altruism. "These individuals want to help society," said Dr. Dwight McKinney, the executive director of clinical pharmacology. The subjects themselves told a different story. "The only reason I came here is to do a study so I can buy me a car and a new pair of shoes," said a twenty-three-year-old former crack addict who had heard about the Lilly clinic on the streets in Nashville. "I'll get a case of Miller and an escort girl and have sex," another subject told the *Journal.* "The girl will cost me $200 an hour."

Unlike many pharmaceutical companies, which contract with university hospitals or contract research organizations to conduct Phase I trials, Lilly had been operating its own testing clinic since 1926. Dr. Leigh Thompson, a former chief scientific officer for Lilly, told the *Journal* that Lilly was already using homeless people as subjects when he arrived at the company in 1982. "We were constantly talking about whether we were exploiting the homeless," he recalled. But he and others felt that the company was offering the subjects a decent bargain. "Providing them with a nice warm bed and good medical care and sending them out drug- and alcohol-free was a positive thing to do." However, the *Journal* noted that Lilly paid subjects the lowest per diem in the business and recruited them from a homeless shelter supported by the Lilly Endowment, a charity funded by Lilly stock. Many of the subjects had alarming stories to tell about their time in the clinic. One said that a Lilly drug had given him a heart problem so bad "they had to put things on my chest to start my heart up again."

Research on human subjects has generated libraries of scholarly commentary. The dominant stream in bioethics sees the crucial issue as informed consent. Can the subject make a free and informed choice about whether to take part in a drug study? Does he know what he is agreeing to do? But a minority opinion sees the issue as one of justice and exploitation. To these scholars, it makes a crucial difference if a subject is sleeping on a hot-air grate and foraging for meals from a dumpster. Poverty, illness, and addiction render subjects vulnerable to exploitation by powerful corporations. And of course, a pharmaceutical company seeking honest moral counsel about testing drugs on homeless alcoholics would get very different answers depending on which ethicists they asked.

After the *Wall Street Journal* story broke, Lilly hired a team of bioethics consultants that included Tom Beauchamp of Georgetown, the coauthor of *Principles of Biomedical Ethics,* perhaps the best-known academic textbook on the subject, and Robert Levine of Yale, the editor of *IRB,* a prominent research ethics journal. Both are scholars squarely in the bioethics mainstream. Beauchamp, in fact, is the coauthor of a notable book on informed consent. What the bioethicists privately advised Lilly to do is unknown, but given their previous writing and ideologies, their published take on the issue was not surprising. In an article in the *Journal of Medicine and Philosophy,* they and their coauthors concluded, "It is not unethical or exploitative to use homeless people in Phase I studies if the system of subject selection is fair, consents are well informed and bona fide, and the risks are not exceptional for the pharmaceutical industry."[16]

It is hard to know if these ethicists were compromised by their payments from Lilly, since their published answer to the problem is consistent with their past writings. There was no dramatic reversal after the Lilly consultation, no inexplicable turnaround. Equally hard to know is whether Lilly picked these particular ethicists because they seemed likely to endorse what the company wanted to do. Yet if a particular ethicist's answer is thoroughly predictable, what exactly is the purpose of hiring the ethicist to say it? Why not simply read what he or she has written?

For critics of corporate consultation, the main reason companies are setting up advisory boards and hiring consultants is damage control. Ethically controversial actions can be defended by saying "We ran it by our ethicists." When scientists at the Jones Institute of Reproductive Medicine found themselves being scrutinized in 2001 after announcing that they had created embryos for research purposes, they told the me-

dia they had consulted with three panels of ethics experts before pro-
ceeding.[17] (They would not name the ethicists, however.) The fact that
the approval of an ethics board counts as a meaningful justification for
controversial actions is testimony to how far the field of bioethics has
risen. What is unclear is whether hired ethicists actually have the power
to stop unethical actions. Do they modify company policy in a meaningful way, or are they hired to make selling easier?

· · ·

Historians quibble about when and where the field of bioethics emerged,
but many observers agree that bioethics is rooted in scandal. In the
United Kingdom the catalyzing event was Maurice Pappworth's 1967
book *Human Guinea Pigs,* which cataloged over two hundred cases of
brazen research abuse, such as drilling holes in patients' skulls in order to study the physiology and injecting patients with malaria parasites
and cancer cells, often without the subjects' knowledge.[18] In New Zealand, the scandal was the "unfortunate experiment" in the 1960s and
1970s at Auckland Women's Hospital, in which women with precancer-
ous cervical abnormalities were studied but not treated for cancer, despite the availability of treatment.[19] Many of these women subsequently
died from cervical cancer. The United States saw an entire catalog of research scandals emerge during this period, the two most notorious of
which occurred at the Willowbrook State Hospital in New York, where
mentally disabled children were injected with the hepatitis virus, and in
Tuskegee, Alabama, where black men with syphilis went untreated for
years after treatment was available.[20]

The 1960s and 1970s were also a time of deeply puzzling moral
dilemmas, many of them raised by new medical technologies: organ
transplantation, ventilators, the artificial heart, genetic engineering, and
in-vitro fertilization. One of the earliest controversies, documented in a
Life cover story by Shana Alexander in 1960, concerned the distribution of
dialysis to patients with failing kidneys at a hospital at the University of
Washington. The decision about which patients should receive dialysis
was made by what came to be known as the "God committee"—a group
of community members who decided, as Alexander put it, who shall live
and who shall die.[21] The development of dialysis itself was not nearly as
ethically controversial as the process by which the decision to allocate
it was made, especially the appeal to the "social worth" of candidates.[22]
The "God committee" had explicitly recommended that patients deemed
more valuable to society should be given preference for dialysis.

In the early days of bioethics, most of the academics who were drawn to these issues came from outside clinical medicine. Many were theologians or scholars in religious studies, such as Paul Ramsey, Joseph Fletcher, and Richard McCormick. Few had any links to organized medicine. The first bioethics think tank, the Hastings Center, was independent of any university or medical school when it was established in 1969 by Dan Callahan, a philosopher, and Willard Gaylin, a psychiatrist. The Kennedy Institute of Ethics was founded at Georgetown University soon afterward, but it was not connected to the medical school. Many of the earliest conversations about bioethics included physicians, but often these were physicians deeply worried about the direction that their profession was taking. In fact, many were sharp critics of medicine— concerned about the way technology was shaping society, skeptical of the research imperative, distrustful of medical authority.

Gradually, however, the shape of bioethics began to change. As it gained a measure of legitimacy, bioethics started to become more tightly incorporated within the structures of medicine itself. Partly this was driven by academic necessity: in the early days many philosophers, lawyers, and religious studies scholars found they had little sense of what actually went on in hospitals and research labs. To write about a critical care unit or an operating room without ever having set foot in one seemed a little like an anthropologist writing about the Trobriand Islanders without ever having left campus. But allowing ethicists on the inside made sense for academic health centers as well. Physicians concerned about the path that medicine was taking felt that ethicists could change the profession's course by teaching ethics to medical students and residents and by making ethics part of hospital culture. And for administrators worried about the threat of external regulation and oversight due to ethical scandals, hiring bioethicists seemed like a way to demonstrate their good intentions.

One notable sign of this change was the emergence in the 1980s of "clinical ethics."[23] Clinical ethicists offered a practical, hands-on service intended to improve patient care. The signature issue of clinical ethics was end-of-life care, and its intellectual center was the University of Chicago, which established its Center for Clinical Medical Ethics in 1984. Whereas academic bioethics had been dominated by theologians and philosophers with the occasional lawyer in the mix, clinical ethics was dominated by physicians. From the start, clinical ethics positioned itself within hospitals. No longer would doctors be forced to listen to the carping and criticism of outsiders; they could do bioethics themselves. And they could do it in the way that they practiced medicine: wearing a white coat, carrying a pager, writing consultation notes in patients' charts. Clinical ethicists set up ethics consultation services on hospital wards, offering moral advice the way a consulting neurosurgeon might recommend a lumbar puncture or a dermatologist might suggest a biopsy.

Another important push came from the federal government. The Human Genome Project was a massive $3 billion program founded in 1990 and headquartered in the Department of Energy and the National Institutes of Health. Headed by the Nobel laureate James Watson (of Watson-and-Crick double-helix fame), the Human Genome Project funded scientific efforts to map the genetic constitution of the human species. Fortunately for bioethicists, the project also set aside 5 percent of its budget for ethical and legal issues. The ELSI (Ethical, Legal and Social Implications) Research Program proved to be a financial windfall. (Arthur Caplan famously called it the "full employment act for bioethicists.") ELSI brought a much wider range of scholars into bioethics: not just geneticists interested in ethics, but also public-health researchers, epidemiologists, and medical sociologists. Indirectly, it also allowed university administrators to fund bioethics programs in the same way as other medical research centers, requiring faculty members to support their own salaries through external grants.

I stumbled into bioethics during this period of the field's transformation. Although I originally trained in medicine, I had moved to the University of Glasgow in Scotland to study philosophy after graduating from medical school in South Carolina. Unlike some doctors, who turn to philosophy in order to get a deeper, richer understanding of medicine, I turned to philosophy mainly because I wanted to escape. I found philosophy a much more congenial place to work: abstract where medicine was concrete, skeptical where medicine was dogmatic and authoritarian. But philosophy was also pretty hard on the wallet, especially if you owed medical-school loans. When I applied for a fellowship at the University of Chicago in 1989, I knew very little about American bioethics and had no idea that Chicago was the center of the budding clinical ethics movement. All I really knew was that the fellowship offered a salary.

A little to my surprise, I found a lot to like. For one thing, the doctors who gravitated toward bioethics tended to be a gentler, more thoughtful breed than their colleagues in the medical mainstream. Many of them had become disillusioned with the hard edges of clinical medicine. More than a few had struggled for years in their own institutions, trying to maneuver ethics into the medical-school curriculum and residency training programs, often volunteering their own time without compensation. The professional atmosphere of bioethics was unexpectedly welcoming, and its gatherings much friendlier than those of philosophy meetings, where public debates could have the feeling of a martial arts cage match. The field was thoroughly interdisciplinary, and many people seemed drawn to it because they felt marginalized in their home disciplines. The conferences often had an atmosphere of refuge, like a club for non-joiners.

Yet bioethics also attracted more than its share of academic entrepreneurs. Many bioethicists seemed just a little too enthusiastic about the position of authority bestowed on them by their titles. Often the most zealous ethicists were the public face of the field, offering glib commentary on television. Some were doctors, but many were also humanities scholars eager to take advantage of the money and prestige that went along with academic medicine. The field also included an unexpectedly high percentage of second-rate scholars. Academic health centers were hiring bioethicists, but the people in charge of hiring were often ill-equipped to make those decisions. Many administrators seemed interested mainly in hiring charismatic spokespeople who would support their mission and generate grant revenue.

In the early days, the primary centers for bioethics were state universities and newly established medical schools. By the 1990s, the elite medical centers had started to join in, establishing their own bioethics programs. Bioethics also started migrating into other centers of medical power. The American Medical Association established a bioethics program. So did the Veterans Administration, NASA, and the National Institutes of Health. President Clinton appointed a National Bioethics Advisory Commission, which was followed by the President's Council on Bioethics. Some ethicists began working in the private sector, in businesses such as pharmaceutical and biotechnology companies and at commercial IRBs. As the status of bioethics began to rise in the outside world, universities began to take notice. University administrators made more high-profile bioethics appointments, sometimes with endowed chairs. Often these appointments were determined not on the basis of the ethicist's scholarship but because he or she had played a prominent role for a professional body or a federal bioethics commission.

By the early 2000s, the figure of the bioethicist had changed. It had become possible for a person to be employed as a bioethicist without ever having worked as a professor, a doctor, a lawyer, a minister, or anything else. The bioethicist was invested with a kind of social authority, partly because of his or her specialized education, but also because of the individual's distinct place in an institution's bureaucracy. The clinical ethicist, for instance, was given authority simply by virtue of the fact that he or she occupied the institutional position of "clinical ethicist," which came with certain trappings (a white coat, an office, a hospital ID, responsibility for certain committees) and a certain amount of deference within the organization. Today many physicians and nurses working in hospitals feel they cannot just ignore the moral advice of the clinical ethicist, even if they believe it is wrong.

Bioethics scholarship also began to change. No longer was the default position of bioethicists a suspicion of medical technology. Human cloning, gene therapy, embryonic stem cell research, cosmetic psychopharmacology: a new generation of ethicists saw the same kind of utopian promise in biotechnology that others saw in the digital revolution. Many ethicists began to press to increase funding for medical research. Some offered wildly enthusiastic predictions about our technology-enhanced future. (In 2003, bioethicist Glenn McGee told the *Philadelphia Inquirer* that a device the size of an iPod would soon give us daily downloads about what to eat and let us have drugs tailor-made for our personal use. "I'm talking five years," he said. [24] In his book *Beyond Genetics*, McGee predicted that "no middle-class suburbanite will be without home DNA analysis in 2010."[25] In 2004, James Hughes forecast that in two decades "transsexuals will be able to have new, fully functional genitalia cloned, grown and transplanted." He also suggested it will be possible to genetically engineer elves, unicorns, and centaurs, although he did not give a timeline for when the technology would be developed.[26]) To some outsiders, it appeared that bioethics had been co-opted by the very institutions it was intended to study. Many observers agreed with sociologist Jonathan Imber when he called bioethics "the public relations division of modern medicine."[27]

One striking example of this transformation came after one of the most notorious research scandals of the 1990s. Jesse Gelsinger was only eighteen years old when he flew from Tucson to Philadelphia to take part in a gene therapy study at the University of Pennsylvania. Gelsinger had been born with ornithine transcarbamylase (OTC) deficiency, a rare metabolic illness that makes it impossible for the liver to clear ammonia from the body. OTC deficiency kills most children shortly after they are born. Gelsinger, however, was a relatively healthy young man. He had a mild form of the disorder, which he had been able to control with drugs and diet. The gene therapy study at Pennsylvania used a modified cold virus to carry corrective genes to the liver, in the hope that they would fix the metabolic deficiency. When the Penn researchers injected Gelsinger with the virus, however, he rapidly went into multisystem organ failure. Within only a few days, he was dead.

Gelsinger's death stunned scientists who had seen gene therapy as an extraordinarily promising area of research. It also shocked many bioethicists. An FDA panel found that Gelsinger should never have been considered for the trial because of the condition of his liver.[28] A lawsuit charged that the Penn researchers had not been completely honest with Gelsinger about the potential risks of the study. The study was also compromised by serious conflicts of interest: the researcher in charge, James Wilson, held a 30 percent controlling interest in Genovo, the biotechnology company that stood to profit from the study.[29] Genovo also provided $4 million a year to the research program Wilson directed, the Institute for Human Gene Therapy. Still another ethical controversy concerned the design of the trial. Most potentially risky trials of new drugs for serious illnesses (such as cancer) are done on the patients most severely affected by the disease and whose prognosis is very poor without any treatment. But because the severely affected patients in the case of OTC deficiency are newborns, unable to give informed consent, the Penn researchers had decided to test the gene therapy on adult patients with mild forms of the disorder, such as Gelsinger. This meant that healthy patients with long lives ahead of them were exposed to the risk of serious injury and death.

Shortly after Gelsinger died, two bioethicists at the University of Pennsylvania, Arthur Caplan and David Magnus, published a newspaper op-ed about the study. Remarkably, they did not criticize the study in any way. Rather, they lamented the fact that Gelsinger's death might slow the pace of medical research by leading to tighter regulation. "We do a disservice to Jesse Gelsinger and others who have been hurt or killed in medical research by simply adding layers of bureaucracy in the path of clinical research," the bioethicists wrote. "If we are not careful we may wind up allowing our collective grief over the death of a young research subject to justify the imposition of bad public policy governing the future of gene therapy."[30]

The op-ed was not widely noticed, yet it represented a remarkable transformation for bioethics. In the 1970s and 1980s bioethicists were often deeply resented by doctors, who regarded them as naïve and arrogant outsiders intruding on the doctors' professional turf. By the mid-1990s, however, bioethicists were demonstrating that they not only did not threaten medicine but also could be loyal members of the medical team. In 1996, Benjamin Freedman, a colleague of mine in the Biomedical Ethics Unit at McGill University, wrote a controversial article called "Where Are the Heroes of Bioethics?"[31] If bioethicists were genuinely speaking their minds about ethical problems in hospitals and research labs, Freedman thought, surely there would be times when they would be punished. Bioethicists critical of unethical practices would lose their jobs, find themselves censured by hospital authorities, and have their tenure applications denied. Yet there seemed to be remarkably few cases, if any, where this had happened. Freedman wondered: what does this say about the direction that bioethics is traveling?

• • •

Not many philosophy professors have the sign CHIEF EXECUTIVE OFFICER on their doors. In fact, the very thought would make many philosophers shudder. But in 1999, after a twenty-year career in academic philosophy, one that had begun with a Rhodes Scholarship at Oxford, Willem Landman became the CEO of the Ethics Institute of South Africa (EthicsSA). EthicsSA is an independent, nonprofit company specializing in medical and business ethics that was started with a $3 million grant from the Merck Company Foundation. When Willem decided to take the job, he was teaching bioethics at the medical school at East Carolina University in North Carolina. He flew to Pretoria to meet the Merck board members. "I'll never forget it," he told me. "I met them all at the Merck offices, and the whole board was there. I remember staying in a hotel, and looking out over the historic union buildings, and I remember wanting to jump out of the window." He pauses a moment and laughs. "I thought: I've made the biggest mistake of my life and I can't reverse it."

Willem is an unpretentious Afrikaner with a dark, self-effacing sense of humor. He carries a slight air of awkwardness about him, maybe because he is too tall to fit comfortably into ordinary-size spaces. He always seems to be about to bump his head on doorjambs and low-hanging ceiling lamps. We met each other in the early 1990s when I was a postdoctoral research fellow at the University of Natal Medical School (now the Nelson Mandela School of Medicine), which trained non-white South Africans to become physicians. Willem was chair of the Department of Philosophy at the University of Western Cape, an institution for "colored" students and during the apartheid era one of the most politically radical universities in South Africa. As a student Willem had been deeply involved in the anti-apartheid movement at Stellenbosch University, an elite Afrikaans school. He was once briefly detained by the police and later refused to accept his PhD in philosophy because of the fact that P.W. Botha, the hard-line, pro-apartheid president, was honorary chancellor of the university. (Botha called him a traitor.) Within minutes of meeting Willem, I felt sure I would like him. He was outspoken and iconoclastic, but with a kind of goofy charm that suggested he did not take himself too seriously.

When Willem made the unlikely step from philosophy professor to CEO, he had no idea what to expect. "I had a very vague notion that I wanted the institute to assist others who have a need for, well, let's call it 'ethics services,'" he says, "where organizations need to make decisions that have an ethical dimension to them, and they need a facility to help them work through these issues. Or where they have a code of ethics, but the thing is just there because it's required, but it's not a living document. I had an idea that I wanted to get involved in that, but I had no idea how anyone would take notice of one person calling himself an ethicist. I had no idea." He also had no immediate way of generating income for the institution, other than the start-up grant from Merck. "It was quite scary knowing that eventually this institute had to be financially self-sufficient. I had no idea how anyone could make money out of ethics," he says. "I took the plunge because I had an entrepreneurial side to me that was never really satisfied in academia. I thought I was just taking salary, and I've never really built something from scratch."

The Ethics Institute of South Africa is one of four ethics organizations Merck has set up in economically emerging countries. (The others are in Turkey, Brazil, and the United Arab Emirates.) Despite his early misgivings, Willem seems relatively pleased with how things have turned out. "My intuitive approach was: let us establish our credibility by doing research projects that had a very strong practical relevance, but practical also in the sense of social issues in South Africa. I thought we would become a brand that people would recognize, and maybe from that, we could develop services that one could sell," he says. Today EthicsSA employs eight people and supports itself largely by providing ethics services to businesses and government offices: delivering lectures, drafting documents, providing consultations, and setting up courses to train company employees in ethics. In exchange for a membership fee, companies are allowed to display the EthicsSA logo on their communications. Although EthicsSA concentrated on medical ethics in the beginning, it now does consultation work for businesses ranging from Amway to the Bank of Nigeria. It also works with pharmaceutical companies, such as AstraZeneca.

After the Vioxx scandal, it might seem awkward to direct an ethics institute that has a Merck logo on its Web site, not unlike working at the Enron Center for Corporate Responsibility or holding the Richard M. Nixon Chair for Ethics in Government. But Willem sees things differently. While he does not condone Merck's actions, neither does he seem overly disturbed by the Vioxx affair. "It might shock you to hear me say this, but that is quite mild in comparison to some of the other clients we're working with," he says. "You're in a sea of bloody immorality in this place." He seems less outraged by the companies he works with than he is by some government offices, yet the institute has not refused to consult for the government, reasoning that the ethicists have a better chance to influence policy by working with the government than by setting themselves apart. Willem says, "Look, if I start distinguishing between organizations that are kosher and I can work with and those that I can't work with, then I won't do any work."

The Merck money is a sore point between Willem and me. It is no secret that I am generally skeptical about industry-funded bioethics. I was surprised that Willem took the job at EthicsSA. For years he and I had joked about the outsize egos of American bioethicists, and when he was considering the EthicsSA job he told me he was embarrassed by the title of CEO. Over the years I have made a point of e-mailing him regularly with news of pharmaceutical industry scandals, often with a snide comment attached. It is testament to his good nature that he has never taken offense.

Willem does admit that there are some companies whose very missions are so unethical that he would refuse to work with them. "I can't imagine dealing with one of these companies that brings out Americans for canned lion hunts," he says. Once, he says, EthicsSA was contacted by the gambling board of South Africa about how to encourage responsible gambling, and the institute turned down the request. It has also terminated or suspended the membership of some companies.

Willem says that Merck has never pressured him to say anything or to hold back in any way. "We are not in the pockets of anybody," he says. "We don't have to play up to any sort of gallery at all. We make our own money, and we do it through consultations and the like, and we say whatever we want to say." Yet Willem seems to know remarkably little about any of the recent controversies concerning the pharmaceutical industry, including the Vioxx scandal. "In a way, I have turned a blind eye to it," he admits. Pharmaceutical industry wrongdoing was never one of his academic interests, even before his current position. Much of his academic writing has been about animal rights. He seems frustrated by the suggestion that he ought to have looked closer at the Vioxx litigation. "Nobody here actually takes any notice of the fact that we are funded by Merck," he says. "I just don't have the resources to go into an endless debate on what the science is, and how the whole risk issue was managed. There are issues of more pressing concern."

EthicsSA is not the only bioethics center to be funded with pharmaceutical industry money, not even in South Africa. The University of the Witwatersrand, in Johannesburg, has established the Steve Biko Centre for Bioethics with money from Pfizer, which funded a four-year bioethics lectureship.[32] Pfizer has also funded a lectureship in medical humanities at University College London.[33] Still more industry-funded programs have been established in the United States and Canada. In the late 1990s the Stanford University Center for Biomedical Ethics funded a program in genetics with a million-dollar gift from the SmithKline Beecham Corporation (now part of GlaxoSmithKline). The Center for Practical Bioethics (formerly the Midwest Bioethics Center) funded a research integrity project with a donation of $587,870 from the Aventis Pharmaceuticals Foundation; it currently lists Purdue Pharma as a corporate donor in the $100,000 to $400,000 range.[34] Seton Hall University has a visiting lectureship in health law that is supported by Merck, as well as a Center for Health and Pharmaceutical Law and Policy that was funded by a five-million-dollar donation from Bristol-Myers Squibb and a two-and-a-half-million-dollar donation from Schering-Plough, among others.[35] Washington and Lee University hosts an annual Johnson and Johnson Law and Medicine Colloquium.[36] The Hastings Center has disclosed recent gifts from Hoffman-La Roche and Purdue Pharma.[37] The University of Toronto houses the Sun Life Chair in Bioethics, funded by an insurance company.[38] The University of Pennsylvania Center for Bioethics has disclosed funding from a whole range of pharmaceutical and biotechnology companies, from Monsanto and Geron to Pfizer, AstraZeneca, and Schering-Plough.

Some of my South African friends point out that it is much easier for the wealthy to say no to industry money than it is for the poor. And it is true that some American bioethics centers have sought out industry funding even when they could easily find money elsewhere. The University of Pennsylvania, for example, is an expensive Ivy League university with medical and business schools that rank among the best in the country. In South Africa, however, where most people still struggle in poverty that is extraordinary even by American standards, funding for ethics is a lot harder to find. When I worked at the University of Natal Medical School, the teaching hospital was located in a converted World War II military barracks, where patients often slept on the floor. My office was in a former animal-care facility that had once been used to house rats, dogs, and baboons. The construction was so haphazard that the roof collapsed one night during a thunderstorm. I can understand how South African ethicists might find pharmaceutical industry money hard to resist. The question is whether the mission of an ethics center is so vitally important that it can survive the conflicts of interest generated by industry funding.

Years ago some colleagues and I helped put together a special issue of the bioethics journal the *Hastings Center Report*.[39] Several of the papers (including my own) expressed worries about the extent to which antidepressants were being prescribed, especially for patients who were not clinically depressed. One paper in particular, titled "Good Science or Good Business?" by David Healy at the University of Wales, was especially critical of the drug industry. Shortly after the essays were published, Eli Lilly, which manufactures Prozac, withdrew its annual gift to the Hastings Center, citing the special issue as its reason. Lilly's yearly check for $25,000 was not especially large by industry standards, but it was the Hastings Center's largest annual corporate donation.

The way bioethicists reacted to Lilly's actions is emblematic of the difficulties raised by corporate money. Some were encouraged by the response of the Hastings Center staff—particularly by the *Report*'s editors, who had published the special issue without regard to Lilly's reaction. We are never hostage to corporate money, these scholars say. We can always turn it down, resign our posts, and do the right thing despite enticements to the contrary. For others, however, the fact that the *Report*'s editors faced such pressure is precisely the problem. An ethicist can bite the hand that feeds it for only so long before the food stops coming.

While it may be difficult to imagine Willem and his colleagues at EthicsSA publicly attacking Merck's marketing practices, it is hard to argue that academic bioethicists have done a lot better. Academic health centers have had their share of scandals, and it is not easy to think of a case where the bioethicists at those institutions have spoken out publicly, even when they have been tenured. It might be a reluctance to jeopardize their funding that keeps these ethicists from speaking out, but it may also be simply that it is uncomfortable to criticize your friends and colleagues. It is a lot easier to reserve your blistering criticism for strangers whom you will never see in person.

As I listen to Willem describe the actual work of EthicsSA, my impression is not that he has gone over to the Dark Side, although it is true that he spends a lot more time these days on airplanes and in television studios. Rather, it sounds as if he has moved into a kind of ethics limbo, where every cubicle is occupied by a minor bureaucrat with glazed eyes working on an ethics code for Amway salesmen. Whether EthicsSA has actually done any good or not in South Africa I can't say. It is entirely possible that they have reduced corruption and that their courses are making South African businesses more ethical places to work. But the job itself sounds like a soul-deadening series of corporate meetings, workshops, and rule-writing exercises. When I say this to Willem, he just laughs, pointing out that it is not terribly different from some academic jobs, which also require a lot of pointless administrative tasks. "We do things at university, and what impact do you have on society?" he says. "I see these guys who teach business ethics at universities. They don't have the vaguest notion of the pressures that you find and the countervailing forces that you have to negotiate once you are in a decision-making position. They have no bloody idea."

Whatever else his new job had done, it has not turned Willem into a cautious, managerial personality. His public comments are often so biting that it is impossible to imagine them coming from an American ethicist. He wields his weekly newspaper column like a nightstick. If anything, his position has given him a public forum that he could not have dreamed of as an ordinary philosophy professor. "We've reached the stage where on every single public issue, I'm asked to comment," he says. His frequent appearances on television and radio would have been impossible, he says, without the money from Merck.

After ten years, however, the job does seem to be grinding him down. There is a world-weary note in his voice when he says will step away from the institute soon. "Everything is so tainted," he says. "Everything is about contacts and about power plays and about positioning yourself and about covering your rear. It's never about just doing something and be damned the consequences, just doing what is right." Willem tells me he plans to head out into the desert soon, in Botswana and Namibia, with his photographic equipment. "The next ten years, I want to spend my time in nature. I can't handle human beings anymore."

•　　•　　•

In March 2009, the U.S. Government Accountability Office (GAO) announced the successful conclusion of a clandestine "sting" operation.[40]

The targets of the sting were institutional review boards (IRBs), the committees responsible for overseeing the ethics of medical research in the United States. Posing as a bogus corporation called Device Med-Systems, the GAO asked three commercial IRBs to review a study of a fictitious substance called Adhesiabloc gel. The supposed purpose of the study was to find out whether Adhesiabloc would prevent surgical adhesions, a side effect of surgery that occurs when scar tissue causes internal organs to bind together. The GAO designed the Adhesiabloc protocol to appear so risky that any reasonable IRB would turn it down. It called for a liter of Adhesiabloc gel to be poured into the abdominal cavity of a patient after surgery, where it would remain for up to five months.

The GAO intentionally kept the three IRBs in the dark about the protocol. It did not give them the results of any animal studies. It did not tell them where the experimental substance was manufactured. It did not reveal where the proposed surgery would take place, or who would perform it. Although the GAO noted that the experimental substance was 2.5 percent propylene glycol, it did not provide any information about the substance's other 97.5 percent. The principal investigator for the study was given a forged medical license from Virginia dated 1990, which meant that even if the license had been legitimate, it would have already expired. The only contact information the GAO included was a P.O. box and a cell phone number. "It's the worst thing I've ever seen," said a reviewer for one of the IRBs. "Doing a major surgery on a patient, and then a mystery guy comes in and dumps a solution in the body? Where's the safety for the patient?" Yet one commercial IRB approved the protocol within a week.[41]

That was Coast IRB, based in Colorado Springs, Colorado. The GAO had good reason to suspect that Coast IRB was not the most rigorous board in the business. Coast had offered pharmaceutical companies coupons, inviting them to "take us for a free test drive" and to "coast through your next study." Of the 356 protocols that Coast reviewed over a five-year period, it rejected only one. It had also posted an advertisement on YouTube featuring a cartoon schooner. People speaking in phony English accents apparently meant to convey sailors' voices narrated the ad: "Cap'n, we've got to find our way out of this fog!" says one. "Ah, thar she blows! The Coast Independent Review Board! With speed, quality, and service, guided by the light of ethics."[42] Despite these tactics (or perhaps because of them), annual revenue for Coast IRB doubled in only four years, reaching $9.3 million in 2008.[43]

On March 26, 2009, the Energy and Commerce Committee of the U.S.

House of Representatives conducted a hearing on the GAO sting opera-tion. [44] One after another, angry members of Congress waved liter bottles of the fake Adhesiabloc, professing outrage that such a bizarre study had been given a stamp of ethical approval. But Dan Dueber, the CEO of Coast IRB, remained defiant. Refusing to admit any flaws whatsoever in the fake Adhesiabloc study, Dueber maintained that the protocol had been thoroughly vetted by his expert reviewers. In fact, it was Coast IRB that had been victimized, Dueber claimed. "Innocent citizens of this country cannot be lawfully defrauded by the government," he told the congressional committee, noting that he had reported the GAO fraud to the appropriate law enforcement officials. [45]

Representatives from the FDA and the Office for Human Research Protections also attended the congressional hearing. To the surprise of everyone there, however, they refused to criticize Coast IRB. Their re-fusal to pass judgment appeared to make members of Congress even angrier. "I'm so mad at the company I can hardly be civil," said Rep. Joe Barton, a Republican from Texas, "but I'm almost as upset with our gov-ernment folks who are supposed to oversee these IRBs. This company has gotten four or five notice letters in the last two to three years and yet they're still in business. And they have the gall to come here and threaten to sue the government!" [46]

IRBs have a unique place in the bioethics universe. They are the clos-est things to a regulatory arm for which bioethicists can claim any credit. Established in the 1970s, IRBs are supposed to provide independent ethi-cal review before a medical research study proceeds. IRBs were set up as an institutional response to the research scandals of the 1960s and 1970s, such as the ones at Tuskegee and Willowbrook. Today it is a rare bioeth-ics course that does not include the ethics of human research, and many bioethicists serve on IRBs at their own institutions. Over the years, re-search ethics has evolved into the most bureaucratic, legalistic subfield of bioethics, spawning its own unique subculture with members that in-clude not just academics but also industry executives, IRB members, and government functionaries, all of whom gather each year at a conference called Public Responsibility in Medicine and Research (PRIM&R).

In the early days, IRBs were mainly volunteer committees made up of clinicians and researchers working in the hospitals and medical schools where studies were being conducted. During the 1990s, however, as drug studies migrated out of academic health centers and into the pri-vate sector, a new type of IRB emerged: independent, for-profit boards that reviewed studies for pharmaceutical companies and other research sponsors in exchange for a fee. This arrangement would prove profitable for both parties. By 2002, more than forty commercial IRBs were operating in the United States with over $60 million in annual revenue.[47] In 2004, Chesapeake IRB, one of the largest commercial IRBs, was named by Deloitte as one of the fastest-growing tech companies in America.[48]

Commercial IRBs have proven controversial, for the obvious reasons. Since they are paid by the companies whose protocols they review, commercial IRBs have a financial interest in keeping their clients happy. They market themselves by promising industry-friendly service and a quick turnaround for reviews. No research sponsor is obligated to stick with a single IRB; if a study is rejected by one commercial IRB as too risky or deceptive, the sponsor can simply send it to other IRBs until it is approved. Proponents of commercial IRBs argue that it is in the interest of research sponsors to obtain a strict review, if only to head off potential litigation later. (In fact, lawsuits about clinical trials are still relatively rare.) However, the costs of delaying a study because of a slow, rigorous ethical review can be considerable. In its "lost schooner" advertisement, Coast IRB told potential customers that a delay of a single day for a fifty-center, Phase III trial could cost a sponsor six million dollars.[49]

Surprisingly, bioethicists have given commercial IRBs a fairly easy ride. Some bioethicists even work for commercial IRBs as reviewers. Goodwyn IRB in Ohio, for example, lists a number of distinguished university-based bioethicists on its review board, even as it markets itself as a "good friend to pharmaceutical manufacturers."[50] Dr. Ezekiel Emanuel, formerly the chief of bioethics at the National Institutes of Health, has been a vocal supporter of commercial IRBs, especially Western IRB in Olympia, Washington. "I think there are a lot of reasons that make Western and a few of the others very good," Emanuel told the President's Council on Bioethics a few years ago. "One is certainly leadership and dedication to doing the right thing, and believing that by doing the right thing, you'll be successful, and in their case profitable."[51]

IRBs themselves are not carefully overseen. There is an accreditation body for IRBs, but accreditation is voluntary. The federal Office for Human Research Protections maintains an IRB registry, but registration for an IRB does not exactly guarantee quality. In fact, the GAO sting operation that sank Coast IRB also targeted the OHRP registration process. GAO staffers were able to register a fake IRB located in Chetesville, Arizona, chaired by a three-legged German shepherd called Truper Dawg, with members named April Phuls, Alan Ruse, and Timothy Wittless.[52]

Part of the reason commercial IRBs have been successful is the fact that university-based IRBs have so many problems of their own. It is probably fair to say that IRBs rank among the most thoroughly despised parts of the academic bureaucracy. Dr. Fredric Coe, a nephrologist at the University of Chicago, calls IRBs a "tedious, time-wasting, work-wasting machine."[53] It is hard not to sympathize. Having a research protocol reviewed by an IRB combines the most unpleasant parts of an IRS audit and an afternoon at the Department of Motor Vehicles. (I say this as a former IRB member at four different institutions who is completely sympathetic to both the mission of IRBs and the thankless work of serving on one. As bad as it may be to spend an afternoon at the DMV, it is even worse to work there full-time.) Yet as scrupulous as IRBs can be, their exacting standards do not extend to their own potential conflicts of interest. A recent survey of academic IRB members found that nearly half had served as consultants to the drug industry.[54]

Many universities have simply given up on running their own IRBs and now outsource their research review to commercial IRBs. This is partly a result of economic pressure. A recent survey found that university IRBs cost an average of nearly $750,000 annually to operate, maxing out at over $4 million a year at the larger, research-intensive universities.[55] Many IRBs have begun charging sponsors for review. At the University of Minnesota, for example, where I work, the IRB charges a fee of $2,500 to review industry-sponsored studies.[56]

Of course, university IRBs are also located within academic health centers that compete with contract research organizations for clinical trials. As a result, university IRBs must review trials quickly to keep sponsors from taking the trials elsewhere. When they review a trial they must also weigh the potential consequences of rejecting it or asking for modifications. If one university IRB has a reputation for turning down a certain kind of trial, the sponsor may decide to take the next trial of that type somewhere else. And if an IRB asks for too many modifications in a trial—too many changes to the consent form, say, or to the number of blood draws or biopsies—then it risks losing the next trial from that sponsor.

When I was a faculty member at McGill University in Montreal, I served on the IRB of a university-affiliated psychiatric hospital. Soon after I joined, I found myself in sharp conflict with many other members over one recurring issue: the use of placebos in psychiatric clinical trials. When a new psychiatric drug looks sufficiently promising to be tried in human subjects, it is ordinarily tested against a control drug. If there is no effective treatment for the illness in question, that control is a placebo. Some subjects get the new drug, others get a placebo, and the researchers measure how the two compare. But if an effective treatment exists for a research subject's illness, ethics requires that the new drug must be tested against it, not against a placebo. The purpose of this rule is to protect subjects from harm. A patient should not get substandard treatment, such as a placebo, simply because he or she has volunteered for a research protocol. Just as a placebo cannot ethically be given to research subjects who have asthma or cancer or heart disease when drugs for their disease are being evaluated, a placebo ought not to be given to patients with, say, acute schizophrenia, even if the subjects consent to the possibility, because the condition can be treated with existing drugs. If an ordinary psychiatrist were to treat schizophrenia with a placebo rather than standard therapy, he or she could be successfully sued for malpractice.

Or so I argued. The board was reviewing industry-sponsored protocols in which some patients who were acutely psychotic—delusional, hallucinating, confused, tortured by their own thoughts—were being given placebos rather than effective treatments, sometimes for periods of up to eight weeks. I cited national and international ethics guidelines, even the university's own guidelines, all of which prohibited the trials. Tables were pounded. Faces turned scarlet. Blood pressures soared. Yet the IRB continued to approve many of the trials, over my objections and those of other members of the committee. The hospital administration eventually dissolved the IRB and reconstituted it with new membership. I was not removed from the IRB, but many of my allies were, and the IRB continued to approve the studies.

The issue was so divisive because so many interests were at stake. First of all, the pharmaceutical industry, which sponsored the trials, had a financial interest in conducting placebo-controlled trials because these usually required fewer subjects than tests with active controls and thus were less expensive. Second, the trials generated much-needed income for the hospital, and possibly also for the researchers themselves. (The IRB was not privy to the financial details of the studies.) And third, many IRB members were hospital psychiatrists who conducted placebo-controlled trials for industry. Other IRB members worked under the administrative authority of senior psychiatrists who were doing this type of research. It would have been very difficult for them to take a moral stand against their department chair or division chief.

Defenders of commercial IRBs point out that whatever their financial conflicts of interest, their members are not mixed up in the kind of personal and administrative entanglements that make university IRBs so fraught. Commercial IRBs may be paid by research sponsors, but they are often located thousands of miles away from research sites, and their members are usually total strangers to any investigator whose research they review. A review from a commercial IRB can be as faceless and anonymous as a passport application. Anonymity is no guarantee of quality, of course, as the GAO sting of Coast IRB showed. But some commercial IRBs have developed a reputation for serious review. The most prominent of these is Western IRB or, as most people call it, WIRB.

•   •   •

WIRB is the largest commercial IRB in the world, overseeing between two thousand and twenty-five hundred new trials a year. It is headquartered in Olympia, Washington, a small city just south of Seattle. Olympia is the state's capital, but it has the feel of a college town, a funky blend of working-class diners, organic hamburger joints, and restored old theaters. The main WIRB campus is located in a quiet Olympia neighborhood set back among gardens and trees and surrounded by a black, wrought-iron fence. The campus feels like a cross between an academic think tank and an upscale summer camp, until you go inside, where the atmosphere turns expensive and corporate. Here are the leather chairs, the conference tables, and the sophisticated AV equipment. Secretaries work busily at computers. The men and women wear name tags and dress in smart suits.

A few years ago I struck up a correspondence with Dr. Angela Bowen, the founder of WIRB, while I was researching an article for the *New Yorker.* I had been critical of for-profit IRBs, including WIRB, in some of my previous articles, and Dr. Bowen had invited me to visit, presumably to correct some of my poor impressions. In June 2009 I decided to take her up on the offer, largely out of curiosity. WIRB is easily the most dominant force in the business, the Google of research oversight; it is the commercial IRB that supporters most often hold up as an example of excellence.

A few days before I was to leave for Olympia, however, I got an e-mail from a woman identifying herself as the in-house counsel for WIRB. "As a course of policy, WIRB requires visitors to sign a confidentiality agreement," said the message. Attached was a copy of the agreement, which I was invited to review. Nervously, I clicked open the attachment. The more I read, the more anxious I became. As I expected, the agreement prohibited me from revealing any information that I might learn about WIRB customers. But it also went much further. In fact, signing the agreement seemed to prohibit me from revealing anything I learned about WIRB on my visit to anyone else, ever. The information that WIRB considered "confidential and proprietary" included any facts concerning its finances, business policies, projects, proposals, regulatory affairs, or production processes. So thorough was the list of things that I was prohibited from discussing that it was hard to think of anything about the visit that I would ever be allowed to mention. The agreement concluded, "I understand that a breach of this Agreement will cause immediate and irreparable harm to WIRB. I understand that my obligation to abide by the terms of this Agreement shall continue indefinitely."

I contacted a reporter who had visited WIRB and asked if he had signed any confidentiality agreement. He said he had not signed anything, adding, "What sense would that make for a journalist?" When I arrived at the WIRB campus the next week and identified myself at the reception desk, a young man presented me with the agreement. When I explained that I was not planning to sign it, he summoned a senior executive, a polite, rather tightly wound lawyer in a dark suit whom I had met briefly several years before at a bioethics conference. As I explained my position the lawyer led me into a private conference room, his face frozen into a polite smile, like a gracious host trying to manage a dinner guest with appallingly bad table manners. Insistently he tried to persuade me to sign modified versions of the agreement, offering various compromises until it became clear that his efforts were futile, after which he settled back in his chair, defeated. I offered to leave, but after some anxious phone calls with other company officials it was decided that my visit could continue as long as I did not sit in on any meetings of their review boards.

The roots of WIRB go back to 1968, several years before the traditional IRB system was put into place, when Dr. Bowen set up a community advisory board to monitor her own research in endocrinology. The company was incorporated in 1977. Today it reviews trials from sponsors in thirty-four countries and has set up review panels in Vancouver, British Columbia, and Santiago, Chile.[57] It has worked with every major pharmaceutical and device manufacturer as well as many biotechnology companies and contract research organizations. WIRB employs over three hundred people and maintains fourteen different review panels, each of which consists of nine standing members as well as alternates. What has given WIRB its credibility among insiders, however, is its work with universities, especially those facing trouble after research scandals. Beginning in 1996, after the unexpected death of a healthy nineteen-year-old student, Nicole Wan, in a clinical trial at the University of Rochester, WIRB has become the commercial IRB of choice for panicked university administrators desperate to sort out their review system. Today WIRB reviews protocols for academic health centers from Johns Hopkins University to the National Cancer Institute.

Its record is not exactly spotless.[58] In the 1990s WIRB gave ethical approval to studies in Los Angeles and Georgia that later turned out to be fraudulent. The Georgia researchers, Richard Borison and Bruce Diamond, made over ten million dollars conducting drug trials in the 1990s, four million of it from schizophrenia studies. To recruit male patients with schizophrenia, Borison and Diamond employed attractive young women and paid them thousands of dollars in recruiting bonuses. One especially successful female recruiter was given a Honda Accord.[59] (In 2005, seven years after Borison was convicted and sentenced to fifteen years in federal prison, Bowen defended her company's oversight of his trials, telling reporters, "I didn't see that there were patient-safety issues.")[60] WIRB was also sued for approving a placebo-controlled study of a Genentech drug called Raptiva. In that study, Bill Hamlet, a patient in North Carolina ill with psoriatic arthritis, claims that he was taken off his regular medications, which had been effective, and given a placebo instead. When Hamlet withdrew from the study six months later, he says his body was covered with bleeding scabs and he was bedridden from his psoriatic arthritis. The lawsuit was settled out of court.[61]

Given the fact that I turned out to be an unpleasant guest in Olympia—underdressed for the visit, unwilling to sign their legal forms, and on the record as a skeptic of commercial IRBs—the WIRB officials proved to be surprisingly congenial hosts. The president of WIRB, Dr. Stephen Rosenfeld, is a hematologist from New York who used to run a clinical center at the NIH. Lanky and bearded, Rosenfeld votes Democratic and drives a Mini, which he used to ferry me across town to the office of Angela Bowen. Dr. Bowen, the founder of WIRB, is a warm, grandmotherly woman with formal manners and a Mississippi accent not very different from mine. (Everyone at WIRB, no matter how senior, refers to her as Dr. Bowen.) When she introduced me to a colleague, she told him, "He's from the South, so don't use too many big words." In fact, almost all the people I met, with the possible exception of the doorkeeping attorney, seemed to be pleasant, well-intentioned types who would not be out of place on a university campus. I felt no trace of the defensiveness and aggression evident in, say, the testimony of Coast CEO Dan Dueber to Congress. The employees seemed genuinely proud of the company and convinced that if I could just see how they operated, I would understand that they sat on the side of the righteous.

There was one embarrassing exception to their openness. Virtually everyone I met appeared happy to talk to me about all manner of topics —the company philosophy, the oversight system, commercial IRBs, the Coast IRB hearings—but whenever I asked a question about finances, lips immediately zipped up tight. Nobody would tell me who had a financial stake in WIRB, who sat on the board of directors, what the company was worth, or how much it earned. Apparently, in the absence of a written promise to keep the information secret, I could not be told anything about the financial status of the company. When I impolitely mentioned that it seemed perverse to set up an oversight system to protect research subjects yet keep information about funding and control of the company secret from the very people being protected, nobody disagreed. But still no one would answer any questions about money.

This may have been because the ownership of WIRB had recently changed. In 2007 a majority stake in WIRB was sold to a private equity firm called Boston Ventures.[62] Boston Ventures is best known for its holdings in the media and entertainment industries. Its portfolio has included such companies as Six Flags Entertainment, American Media, Inc. (the publisher of the *National Enquirer*), and Petty Holdings, the NASCAR racing organization. (It also has holdings in the medical communications company Oakstone Publishing.) According to publicly available reports, the reason for the sale was to prepare for Dr. Bowen's retirement as president. The terms of the sale were not revealed, but three executives from Boston Ventures were appointed to the WIRB board of directors. Bowen retired as president of WIRB the next year, but has remained as chair of the board, and Rosenfeld was hired as the new president.[63]

Nothing about Boston Ventures was mentioned during my visit. What was mentioned, several times, was the general sense of disappointment at WIRB that I would not be "going to board." *Going to board* was their term for the review board meetings, where panel members review actual studies, and which I could not observe without signing a confidentiality agreement. The obsession with confidentiality seemed a little odd to me; I have spent many years serving on university and hospital IRBs, reviewing countless drug company protocols, and I have never been asked to sign a confidentiality agreement. In fact, in some countries, IRB meetings are public and can be attended by anyone who wishes. I could not really imagine that the WIRB board meetings could be all that different from the IRB meetings I had seen before, yet the WIRB executives seemed convinced that if I would just sign the agreement and see how they reviewed protocols, I would be very impressed.

It took a while for me to see just why the confidentiality agreement was so important. WIRB needed for me to remain silent about the specific way they reviewed protocols, because these review methods were themselves proprietary information. Whatever WIRB panel members did in those board meetings, it would be treated as a trade secret. At a university, of course, this obsession with secrecy would be utterly foreign. When I worked at McGill, for instance, the Biomedical Ethics Unit organized conference days where the various hospital IRBs would share with one another their methods of reviewing protocols so that each IRB could learn from the others and improve its practices. In the world of commercial IRBs, however, sharing this kind of information might put you at a competitive disadvantage.

As I drove away from the WIRB campus, it struck me that this obsession with secrecy was the hidden perversity of putting research oversight into the marketplace. Once such competitive pressures are instituted, there is no reason for any commercial IRB to share techniques to improve oversight. In fact, there is every reason *not* to share, because each commercial IRB has a competitive interest in the failure of other IRBs. This competitive interest is built into the system. Even if the members of any given commercial IRB sincerely want to protect the research subjects they oversee, they do not have any financial reason to want other IRBs to protect them, because every IRB that fails represents a potential business opportunity for the ones left standing.

•   •   •

On the Web site of the Washington Speakers Bureau is a video clip of Arthur Caplan, the director of the Center for Bioethics at the University of Pennsylvania.[64] Caplan has developed a unique niche in bioethics; he is a critic of pharmaceutical industry gifts and payments to doctors but works as a paid consultant to industry himself. "Even small gifts influence behavior," Caplan told the *Minneapolis Star Tribune* in 2008.[65] Industry payments to doctors are "too damn lucrative to believe anyone can resist," Caplan said to the *New York Times,* noting that payments will distort people's judgment.[66] Yet Caplan has consulted for companies such as Pfizer, DuPont, and Celera, and the University of Pennsylvania Center for Bioethics has disclosed funding from dozens of pharmaceutical and health-care corporations.

In the video Caplan describes his work as a consultant for Pfizer in the 1990s, when the company was deciding how to market Viagra, its drug for erectile dysfunction. "Pfizer was terrified," says Caplan. "They thought, 'If we come out with this pill, people are going to attack us for promoting sex.'" Caplan points out that Pfizer had not been in the business of reproductive medicine or sexual health. "They were terrified that this drug could get them in trouble on ethics grounds—that people would call them from churches and other organizations and say, 'Why are you promoting this kind of thing?'" They needed to know "How do you advertise this thing so that you can say to people, 'Look this treats a serious problem. It's not just a joke, or a lark.'"

Caplan goes on to explain how he helped Pfizer as a bioethicist. "At meeting after meeting we were trying to figure out who might step forward and say: they had a problem in the sexual function area; they were happy to have the pill help them; it was a disease; erectile dysfunction would be seen as a disease; and say that this is something they used within their marriage, and it was a good thing," says Caplan. "I suggested that what they needed was a spokesperson who would stand for integrity, and who would never be confused for someone who was just there as a sex object. And so I invented Bob Dole."

Bob Dole, of course, is the former Kansas senator and Republican presidential candidate who endorsed Viagra in television advertisements during the late 1990s. Dole's image as an elderly, serious-minded public figure—the polar opposite of the sexually adventurous demographic that came to embrace Viagra a few years later—helped brand the drug as a legitimate treatment for a medical disorder. Caplan praises Pfizer for blending good bioethics with good marketing. "So that's how they handled the ethical challenge," he says. "They thought about it ahead of time, it was all a part of their marketing campaign; they never made a move without being sure they were talking about the disease and what was going on."

Caplan's work for Pfizer is emblematic of a certain vision of bioethics: the bioethicist's desire to be the power behind the throne, the one whispering in the king's ear. First you must establish a presence in the corridors of power, then you work carefully and judiciously to shape the opinions of the people in charge. It is not an unreasonable aspiration, of course. Yet sometimes the king turns out to be venal, greedy, or corrupt, and when that happens, the line between advice and complicity is blurred. When Caplan advises Pfizer to hire a figure like Bob Dole, for example, it sounds less like sorting out an ethical dilemma and more like an effort to devise a better marketing campaign. What does it say about bioethics when the ethicist is indistinguishable from the public relations counsel?

Critics of industry-funded bioethics usually describe the issue as a conflict of interest, pointing out that bioethicists have other roles in which they are presumed to have a measure of distance from the pharmaceutical industry. Bioethicists teach ethics to college students, for example, who generally do not suspect that the professor may be getting a paycheck from the very corporations whose actions and policies they are discussing in class. But a larger question concerns the direction of bioethics as a field. As bioethics has matured, its practitioners have aspired to a kind of professional expertise. Bioethicists have gained recognition largely by carving out roles as trusted advisers. But embracing the role of trusted adviser means forgoing other potential roles, such as that of the critic. It means giving up on pressuring institutions from the outside, in the manner of investigative reporters. As bioethicists seek to become trusted advisers, rather than gadflies or watchdogs, it will not be surprising if they slowly come to resemble the people they are trusted to advise. And when that happens, moral compromise will be unnecessary, because there will be little left to compromise.

Ken De Ville, an attorney and historian of medicine at East Carolina University, wonders whether bioethics will continue to be an enterprise worth pursuing once it is thoroughly infused with corporate money. "If ethicists are transformed into a bunch of corporate shills who exist only to serve the machine," he asks, "where is the honor in taking part?" Of course, De Ville's comment presumes that there is a distinction between honor and serving the machine. Once the very discipline of bioethics is itself a part of the machine, service is an honor. Laurie Zoloth, the former president of the American Society for Bioethics and Humanities, has written that the real temptations of industry associations are not financial but in the honor and status of corporate consultancies. If she is right and advising a corporation is an honor, then bioethicists have already made the shift from outsider to insider, from critic of the machine to loyal servant.

In recent years, the reputation of the pharmaceutical industry has taken a beating. Profits have fallen off; litigation has risen; and Senator Grassley's investigations have ensured a constant stream of poor publicity. From 1997 to 2005, according to Harris Polls, the public approval rating of the pharmaceutical industry dropped from 80 percent to 9 percent, putting its reputation below every other major business except oil and tobacco companies.[67] Prominent physicians have relentlessly attacked industry practices; several former thought leaders have publicly recanted their work. Yet it is still unclear whether bioethicists are willing to cut their industry ties. If anything, many top bioethicists appear to be ramping up their consulting work.

A few years ago I was invited to give a talk about the pharmaceutical industry at a prominent academic health center. At that point I had written several disapproving articles about pharma-funded bioethics, and my presentation included some pointed criticism. The colleague who invited me appeared to share my views. As I was standing next to the lectern, waiting to be introduced, he leaned over to me and whispered, "Do you mind if I thank Janssen Pharmaceuticals for sponsoring your presentation?"

CODA

NOT LONG AGO, as I was trying to finish this book, I got an unusual speaking invitation. It was from the Turkish Psychiatric Association. They were organizing their Forty-fourth National Congress, and they were planning it around the themes of (1) ethics and (2) anxiety disorders. The conference planners had gotten my name from a mutual friend and they wanted me to give a keynote address. I had not been to Turkey in over twenty years, but the Turks I had met back then were extraordinarily hospitable. I told the conference planners yes, I'd love to come.

I am not quite sure what I expected, but nothing from my previous trip really prepared me for the conference venue. The World of Wonders (WOW) Kremlin Palace is a luxury beach resort on the Aegean Sea that is apparently designed to replicate the experience of a visit to Moscow's Red Square under the influence of psychedelic drugs. It appears to cater especially to wealthy Russians. Not only does the resort include a scale replica of St. Basil's Cathedral, it also has a water park, bumper cars, Jet Skis, trampolines, a lagoon-size swimming pool, and a pancake tent. Guests are invited to dance in a replica of the Senate Building, which has been transformed into a disco decorated with Cubist murals; afterward, they can enjoy a Turkish bath in the Palace of Facets or, inexplicably, indulge in an enchilada at the El Sombrero Mexican Restaurant. The hotel lobby, which was modeled on the State History Museum, was decorated in nineteenth-century style: marble floors, pillars, and iron chandeliers, with faux–old masters European paintings on the walls. At the bottom of the escalator was a giant reproduction of the School of Athens; at the top was an enormous Turkish flag. An oversize gold bust of Ataturk jutted out of the wall next to the check-in desk. The effect was a little like that of the giant talking head in *The Wizard of Oz*.

I arrived in Antalya in the morning and wandered around the WOW Kremlin Palace, slightly dazed and jet-lagged. The surreal vibe of the place was heightened by the crowd of Turkish psychiatrists milling around the lobby, many of whom were dressed in expensive suits and pulling tiny blue tote bags on wheels. The wheeled bags had been distributed by the conference organizers; they were the rare item that did not carry a mark of industry sponsorship. Everything else seemed to be branded: the flat-screen televisions, the banners on the walls, and, most obviously, the pharmaceutical display hall where drug reps dispensed brochures, trinkets, and cappuccino. Dinner was served in a vast dining hall where a white-suited man with a long paddle pulled Turkish flatbread out of a baker's oven. Under an aquarium sat a table of salads decorated with plaster statues in an aquatic theme, including an ornately constructed pirate ship and a semi-pornographic mermaid whose scales were draped with Christmas lights and whose large, bare breasts appeared to be the product of silicone implants. Every table exhibited a flag bearing the name of a popular antidepressant.

Over-the-top marketing displays used to be a staple of medical conferences, but these days they are frowned upon, at least in America. Tote bags and cappuccino are seen as temptations for the greedy and craven. But I have to confess that the WOW Kremlin Palace did not feel all that tempting. It just seemed baffling. I wondered how I was supposed to react. Was this place built to be taken seriously? Or was it all supposed to be ironic and amusingly excessive, like the fake Sphinx in Las Vegas? My disorientation was intensified by the fact that I don't speak any Turkish. The last time I was in Turkey I had driven around the country in a battered Volkswagen with my wife, living out of a backpack. Away from the beach resorts and the wealthy tourists, Turkey can seem like a glimpse into another century, an age of wood smoke and donkey carts. What exactly do the Turks themselves make of the WOW Kremlin Palace? When a platinum blond woman in a bikini and high heels walked past, her arm linked with an aging male companion's, was I supposed to think, *Hotel guest?* or *Russian prostitute?*

We have gotten so accustomed to the notion of prescription drugs as a commodity, an item to be priced, sold, and advertised, that it is hard to imagine that things could be another way. It all seems perfectly ordinary. Yet somehow, marketing the drugs at a luxury resort at the margins of the developing world feels slightly unsettling, like passing a homeless person on the way into an expensive restaurant. Prescription drugs may be a market commodity, but were they really meant to be a consumer good? Prescription drugs fill genuine human needs, or at least they are supposed to. It is only when you are faced with genuinely needy people that the prescription-drug marketplace begins to seem perverse.

I delivered my lecture on ethics and the pharmaceutical industry the next morning. Although the lecture was billed as a plenary session, the hall was sparsely populated, and nobody seemed terribly interested. I felt like a preacher delivering a sermon to a congregation of sleeping Presbyterians. The audience listened through headphones to a simultaneous translation of my talk while staring blankly into the distance. When I finished, there was a long silence, then polite applause and more silence. The moderator asked for questions. After more long silence, an audience member finally figured out something to ask. Additional silence followed. Then I was given a plaque.

That evening, I took a walk around the resort with Yasemin Oguz, a Turkish physician and ethicist. Yasemin and I had become friends during a year she spent on sabbatical in Minnesota. We walked down to the water, next to the catamaran and the Jet Skis, and looked back at the replica of St. Basil's Cathedral, which was glowing against the night sky. I remarked that it seemed ironic that the Kremlin, a place that I associate so closely with Cold War communism, should be so fully transformed to the purposes of consumer capitalism. But Yasemin quickly corrected me. The Kremlin Palace was built by the czars, she pointed out. It is not a symbol of communism. It is a symbol of empire.

ACKNOWLEDGMENTS

I T MIGHT HAVE BEEN POSSIBLE to write this book without spending a year at the Institute for Advanced Study in Princeton, but it would not have been nearly as much fun. When Cliff Geertz invited me to help him organize a bioethics seminar in the School of Social Science in 2003, I had no idea what an extraordinary year I was in for. I am deeply indebted to the School of Social Science for hosting me and my family, and to all the friends and colleagues who made it such a memorable year. I am also grateful to the Bioethics Centre at the University of Otago in Dunedin, New Zealand, my home away from home, for welcoming me back for another visit in 2007. As soon as my family and I leave Dunedin, we begin plotting a way to go back.

The University of Sydney awarded me an International Visiting Research Fellowship in 2007, which allowed me to spend three weeks with my friends and colleagues at the Centre for Values, Ethics and Law in Medicine. My friends at the University of Cape Town Bioethics Centre hosted me for a short sabbatical visit in 2008. I appreciate the warmth and hospitality shown to me in both places. I am also grateful to the National Library of Medicine, part of the National Institutes of Health, which supported my work for this book with a grant for Ethics and Pharmaceutical Marketing (5-G13-LM008916-03). The University of Minnesota Graduate School made a number of the interviews possible by awarding me a Grant in Aid of Research, Artistry and Scholarship. The *Atlantic Monthly* published a short version of chapter 3 under the title "The Drug Pushers," and the *New Yorker* published a version of chapter 1 under the title "Guinea-Pigging." I have been writing about bioethicists and the pharmaceutical industry since 2001, and assorted pieces of chapters 4 and 6 have appeared in *Slate*, the *American Prospect, Dissent*, and the *Cambridge Quarterly of Healthcare Ethics.*

My editor, Helene Atwan, has been exceptionally generous with her time and enthusiastic about the manuscript from the start. My literary agent, Andrew Blauner, has been, as always, a pleasure to work with. Of the many friends and colleagues who have helped me with the ideas in the book, special thanks go to Amy Snow Landa, Bob Helms, Trudo Lemmens, Ken De Ville, Michael Oldani, Joel Roselin, Adriane Fugh-Berman, Liz Woeckner, David Healy, Alastair Matheson, Steve Miles, and Leigh Turner.

There are not many parts of this book that I have not discussed at some point with my father, Bruce Elliott, who is a family physician, and my brother, Hal Elliott, who is a psychiatrist. I would not want to saddle either of them with responsibility for what is in the book, but I cannot imagine having written it without them. The same is true of my wife, Ina, and my children, Crawford, Martha, and Lyle, who have lived through the writing of this book with me and who have tolerated my enthusiasms and obsessions with remarkable patience.

NOTES

INTRODUCTION

1. http://money.cnn.com/magazines/fortune/fortune500/2008/performers/industries/profits/.

CHAPTER ONE: THE GUINEA PIGS

1. Robert Steinbrook, "Gag Clauses in Clinical-Trial Agreements," *New England Journal of Medicine* 352 (2005): 2160–62.

2. Office of Inspector General, Department of Health and Human Services, "Recruiting Human Subjects: Pressures in Industry-Sponsored Clinical Research," Washington, DC, June 13, 2000, http://oig.hhs.gov/oei/reports/oei-01-97-00195.pdf.

3. David Evans, Michael Smith, and Liz Willen, "Big Pharma's Shameful Secret," *Bloomberg Markets* 14 (2005): 36–62, http://dcscience.net/pharma-bloomberg.pdf.http://www.plosmedicine.org/article/findArticle.action?author=Evans&title=Big%20pharma%27s%20shameful%20secret.

4. "PharmaNet Settles Lawsuit for $28.5 Mln," Reuters, August 1, 2007, http://www.reuters.com/article/marketsNews/idUSWEN003420070802.

5. Laurie Cohen, "To Screen New Drugs for Safety, Lilly Pays Homeless Alcoholics," *Wall Street Journal*, November 14, 1996.

6. Trudo Lemmens, "Ethics Review for Sale? Conflict of Interest and Commercial Research Review Boards," *Milbank Quarterly* 78 (2000): 547–84.

7. Office of Inspector General, Department of Health and Human Services, "The Food and Drug Administration's Oversight of Clinical Trials," Washington, DC, September 2007, ii.

8. Gardiner Harris, "Report Assails FDA Oversight of Clinical Trials," *New York Times*, September 28, 2007, http://www.nytimes.com/2007/09/28/health/policy/28fda.html?ex=1348718400&en=30b7a25ac3835517&ei=5124&partner=permalink&exprod=permalink.

9. "Food and Drug Administration's Oversight," ii.

10. Elizabeth Rosenthal, "When Drug Trials Go Horribly Wrong," *New York Times*, April 27, 2006, http://www.nytimes.com/2006/04/07/world/europe/07

iht-drug.html?_r=1. See also Alastair J. J. Wood and Janet Darbyshire, "Injury to Research Volunteers: The Clinical-Research Nightmare," *New England Journal of Medicine* 354(2006): 1869–71.

11. Jeanne Lenzer, "Drug Secrets: What the FDA Isn't Telling," *Slate,* September 27, 2005; online at http://www.slate.com/id/2126918/. See also Gardiner Harris, "Student, 19, in Trial of New Antidepressant Commits Suicide," *New York Times,* February 12, 2004.

12. David Evans, "SFBC Drug Testers Have Tuberculosis after Exposure at Centre," *Bloomberg News,* December 15, 2005, http://www.bloomberg.com/apps/news?pid=10000039&sid=a90OZzPRlkaE&refer=columnist_evans.

13. Robert Whitaker, "Lure of Riches Fuels Testing," *Boston Globe,* November 17, 1998.

14. Gardiner Harris and Janet Roberts, "After Sanctions, Doctors Get Drug Company Pay," *New York Times,* June 3, 2007.

15. Kenneth Getz, "Industry Trials Poised to Win Back Academia," *Applied Clinical Trials* (April 2007): 35–38, http://appliedclinicaltrialsonline.findpharma.com/appliedclinicaltrials/article/articleDetail.jsp?id=416536.

16. Anna Wilde Mathews, "Infected Data: Fraud, Errors Taint Key Study of Widely Used Sanofi Drug," *Wall Street Journal,* May 1, 2006.

17. Sonia Shah, *The Body Hunters: How the Drug Industry Tests Its Products on the World's Poorest Patients* (New York: New Press, 2006).

18. Adriana Petryna, *When Experiments Travel: Clinical Trials and the Global Search for Human Subjects* (Princeton, NJ: Princeton University Press, 2009), 13.

19. George Annas, "Globalized Clinical Trials and Informed Consent," *New England Journal of Medicine* 360 (2009): 2050–53. See also Joe Stephens, "Where Profits and Lives Hang in Balance," *Washington Post,* December 17, 2000.

20. In 1999, Trovan was withdrawn from the market in the United States because of its liver toxicity.

21. Marcia Angell, "Industry-Sponsored Clinical Research: A Broken System," *Journal of the American Medical Association* 300 (2008): 1069–71.

22. The exclusion criteria for studies stipulate that patients at risk of suicide should not be enrolled, but they do not mention anything about patients who are homicidal or at risk of violence to others.

23. Joseph P. McEvoy et al., "Efficacy and Tolerability of Olanzapine, Quetiapine, and Risperidone in the Treatment of Early Psychosis: A Randomized, Double-Blind 52-Week Comparison," *American Journal of Psychiatry* 164 (2007): 1050–60.

24. Duff Wilson, "AstraZeneca Pays Millions to Settle Seroquel Cases," *New York Times,* October 30, 2009, http://www.nytimes.com/2009/10/30/business/30drug.html.

25. Maura Lerner and Janet Moore, "Once Secret Drug Company Documents Put U on the Spot," *Minneapolis Star Tribune,* March 13, 2009, http://www.startribune.com/41470522.html?elr=KArksD:aDyaEP:kD:aUbP:P:Q_V_MPQLa7PYDUiD3aPc:_Yyc:aU7DYaGEP7vDEh7P:DiUs.

26. Philip J. Hilts, *Protecting America's Health: The FDA, Business, and One Hundred Years of Regulation* (New York: Alfred A. Knopf, 2003), 39–43. See also Carol Lewis, "The Poison Squad and the Advent of Food and Drug Regulation," *U.S. Food and Drug Administration Consumer Magazine* (November–December 2002): 1–15, http://www.toxicology.org/gp/21_PoisonSquadFDA.pdf.

27. Hilts, *America's Health*, 42–43.

28. Todd Tucker, *The Great Starvation Experiment: The Heroic Men Who Starved So That Millions Could Live* (New York: Free Press, 2006).

29. Bob Helms, ed., *Guinea Pig Zero: An Anthology of the Journal for Human Research Subjects* (New Orleans: Garrett County Press, 2002), 36.

30. Robert Steinbrook, "Compensation for Injured Trial Subjects," *New England Journal of Medicine* 354 (2006): 1871–73.

31. Michael Smith and David Evans, "Three Drug Testers Claim SFBC Threatened Them," *Seattle Times*, November 20, 2005; online at http://seattletimes.nw source.com/html/businesstechnology/2002634562_testers20.html.

CHAPTER TWO: THE GHOSTS

1. *ACCME Annual Report Data 2008*, Accreditation Council for Continuing Medical Education, http://www.accme.org/dir_docs/doc_upload/1f8dc476–246a -4e8e-91d3-d24ff2f5bfec_uploaddocument.pdf.

2. Arnold S. Relman, "Separating Continuing Medical Education from Pharmaceutical Marketing," *Journal of the American Medical Association* 285 (2001): 2009–12.

3. Robert Steinbrook, "Financial Support of Continuing Medical Education," *Journal of the American Medical Association* 299 (2008): 1060–62.

4. Society for Academic Continuing Medical Education, "Academic CME in North America: The 2008 AAMC/SACME Survey," Association of American Medical Colleges 2009, http://www.sacme.org/site/sacme/assets/pdf/2008_CME _Report.pdf.

5. See the advertisement for Helix Medical Communications in *PharmaVOICE* (March 2007): 31. For more on publication planning, see Elizabeth Pena Villarroel, "Master Plan: The Making of a Successful Publication Strategy," *PharmaVOICE* (March 2007): 28–34; and Sergio Sismondo, "Ghosts in the Machine: Publication Planning in the Medical Sciences," *Social Studies of Science* 39 (2009): 171–98.

6. Anna Wilde Matthews, "Ghost Story: At Medical Journals, Writers Paid by Industry Play Big Role," *Wall Street Journal*, December 13, 2005.

7. American Medical Writers Association Salary Survey 2007, http://www .amwa.org/default.asp?id=196 (available to members only).

8. Barton Moffatt and Carl Elliott, "Ghost Marketing: Pharmaceutical Companies and Ghostwritten Journal Articles," *Perspectives in Biology and Medicine* 50 (2007): 18–31; Sergio Sismondo, "Ghost Management: How Much of the Medical Literature Is Shaped Behind the Scenes by the Pharmaceutical Industry?" *PLoS Medicine* 4 (2007): e286. doi:10.1371/journal.pmed.0040286.

9. Annette Flanagin et al., "Honorary Authors and Ghost Authors in Peer-Reviewed Medical Journals," *Journal of the American Medical Association* 280 (1998): 222–24.

10. At a medical conference in September 2009, some of the same authors from the *JAMA* study presented a similar study that found roughly comparable figures. See Duff Wilson and Natasha Singer, "Ghostwriting Is Called Rife in Medical Journals," *New York Times*, September 10, 2009, http://www.nytimes .com/2009/09/11/business/11ghost.html?_r=1&ref=health.

11. David Healy and Dinah Cattell, "Interface Between Authorship, Industry

and Science in the Domain of Therapeutics," *British Journal of Psychiatry* 183 (2003): 22–27.

12. The marketing document, which was uncovered by a Senate Finance Committee investigation, is available online at http://www.nytimes.com/packages/pdf/politics/20090831MEDICARE/20090831_MEDICARE.pdf. James Edwards of BNET Pharma has a blog post on the document at http://industry.bnet.com/pharma/10004081/forests-lexapro-ghostwriting-budget-was-100k-emory-on -the-payroll/.

13. Natasha Singer, "Medical Papers by Ghostwriters Pushed Therapy," *New York Times*, August 4, 2009, http://www.nytimes.com/2009/08/05/health/research/05ghost.html.

14. Elizabeth Lopatto, Jef Feeley, and Margaret Cronin Fisk, "Lilly 'Ghostwrote' Articles to Market Drug, Files Say," *Bloomberg News*, June 11, 2009, http://www.bloomberg.com/apps/news?pid=20601087&sid=a6yFu_t9NyTY&loc=inter stitialskip.

15. Alison Bass, *Side Effects: A Prosecutor, a Whistleblower, and a Bestselling Antidepressant on Trial* (Chapel Hill, NC: Algonquin Books, 2008), 197.

16. Matthew Perrone, "Glaxo Used Ghostwriting Program to Promote Paxil," Associated Press, August 19, 2009, http://abcnews.go.com/Health/Business/wire Story?id=8366574.

17. Harry Sweeney, "Letter to the Editor: Pharma PR or Medical Education," *Hastings Center Report* 35 (2005): 4.

18. S. N. Goodman et al., "What Are the Factors Determining Authorship and the Order of the Authors' Names? A Study among Authors of the *Nederlands Tijdschrift voor Geneeskunde* (*Dutch Journal of Medicine*)," *Journal of the American Medical Association* 280 (1998): 217–18.

19. The American Medical Writers Association also makes this distinction. See http://www.amwa.org/default.asp?id=466.

20. Steven Shapin, *A Social History of Truth: Civility and Science in Seventeenth-Century England* (Chicago: University of Chicago Press, 1995), 94.

21. Richard Horton, "The Dawn of McScience," *New York Review of Books* 51 (2004): 7–9.

22. I have changed the details about this drug in order to disguise it.

23. Adriane Fugh-Berman, "The Corporate Co-Author," *Journal of General Internal Medicine* 20 (2005): 546–48. See also Adriane Fugh-Berman, "Not in My Name," *Guardian*, April 21, 2005.

24. Adriane Fugh-Berman et al., "Advertising in Medical Journals: Should Current Practices Change?" *PLoS Medicine* 3 (2006): e130. doi:10.1371/journal .pmed.0030130.

25. Richard Smith, *The Trouble with Medical Journals* (London: Royal Society of Medicine Press, 2006), 211.

26. The Wiley Blackwell 2010 journals price list is at http://www3.interscience .wiley.com/aboutus/institutionalCustomers.html#ppv-articleselect.

27. The Elsevier price list for 2010 is at http://www.elsevier.com/wps/find/journalpricing.cws_home/2010subscrippricelistlibr/description.

28. The Springer price list is at http://www.springer.com/librarians/price +lists?SGWID=0-40585-0-0-0.

29. Smith, *Trouble with Medical Journals*, 266.

30. Lawrence Altman, "Inside Medical Journals, a Rising Quest for Profits," *New York Times*, August 24, 1999, http://www.nytimes.com/1999/08/24/health/the-doctor-s-world-inside-medical-journals-a-rising-quest-for-profits.html.

31. David Armstrong, "The *New England Journal* Missed Warning Signs," *Wall Street Journal*, May 15, 2006 (reprinted in the *Pittsburgh Post-Gazette* at http://www.post-gazette.com/pg/06135/690336-114.stm).

32. Mildred Cho and Lisa Bero, "The Quality of Drug Studies Published in Symposium Proceedings," *Annals of Internal Medicine* 124 (1996): 485–89.

33. Bob Grant, "Elsevier Published Six Fake Journals," *Scientist*, May 7, 2009, http://www.the-scientist.com/templates/trackable/display/blog.jsp?type=blog&o_url=blog/display/55679&id=55679. See also Bob Grant, "Merck Published Fake Journal," *Scientist*, April 30, 2009, http://www.the-scientist.com/blog/display/55671/.

34. Philip J. Hilts, *Protecting America's Health: The FDA, Business, and One Hundred Years of Regulation* (New York: Alfred A. Knopf, 2003). This entire account of the thalidomide episode comes from Hilts.

35. Ibid., 158.

36. A brochure given to drug reps said they were "to contact teaching hospitals . . . for the purpose of selling them on Kevadon [thalidomide] and providing them with a clinical supply."

37. The head of the clinical research section wrote in a memo, "Sooner or later we will not be able to stop publication of the side effects of Contergan [thalidomide]. We are therefore anxious to get as many positive pieces of work as possible." See Hilts, *Protecting America's Health*, 360.

38. R. O. Nulsen, "Trial of Thalidomide in Insomnia Associated with the Third Trimester," *American Journal of Obstetrics and Gynecology* 81 (1961): 1245–48.

39. Hilts, *Protecting America's Health*, 151.

40. *Morbidity and Mortality Weekly Report* 46 (1997): 1061–66.

41. Alicia Mundy, *Dispensing with the Truth* (New York: St. Martin's Press, 2001), 159, 181–82.

42. Ibid, 9.

43. Charles Ornstein, "Fen-Phen Maker Accused of Funding Journal Articles," *Dallas Morning News*, May 23, 1999. One draft article included a sentence that read: "Individual case reports also suggest a link between dexfenfluramine and primary pulmonary hypertension." Wyeth had Excerpta delete it.

44. Ibid. See also Mundy, *Dispensing with the Truth*, 164.

45. Mundy, *Dispensing with the Truth*, 79–80.

46. JoAnn E. Manson and Gerald A. Faich, "Pharmacotherapy for Obesity—Do the Benefits Outweigh the Risks?" *New England Journal of Medicine* 335 (1996): 659–60. See also Marcia Angell and Jerome Kassirer, "Editorials and Conflicts of Interest," *New England Journal of Medicine* 335 (1996): 1055–56, and Mundy, *Dispensing with the Truth*, 81, 121–25.

47. Mundy, *Dispensing with the Truth*, 115.

48. Ibid., 119.

49. Ibid., 122–23.

50. Ibid., 116–19.

CHAPTER THREE: THE DETAIL MEN

1. Michael Millenson and Mervin Shalowitz, "Getting Doctors to Say Yes to Drugs: The Cost and Quality Impact of Drug Company Marketing to Physicians," Blue Cross and Blue Shield Association of America, 2003. See also Adriane Fugh-Berman and Shahram Ahari, "Following the Script: How Drug Reps Make Friends and Influence Doctors," PLoS Medicine 4 (2007): e150. doi: 10.1371/journal .pmed.0040150.

2. Michele Goldberg, Tiffany Mortellito, and Bob Davenport, "PE's Annual Sales and Marketing Employment Survey: The Big Squeeze," Pharmaceutical Executive 24 (2004): 40–45, http://www.pharmexec.com/pharmexec/article/article Detail.jsp?id=80921.

3. Milton Liebman, "The Right Media Mix is the Key to Maximizing ROI," Medical Marketing & Media 36 (2001): 92–95.

4. John George, "Secret of Astra Merck," Philadelphia Business Journal, July 25, 1997.

5. "Ulcer Drug Prilosec Tops $5 Billion in Worldwide Sales, Leading the Industry," Associated Press, February 17, 1999.

6. Matthew Herper, "Fight over $6 Billion Drug Begins," Forbes.com, December 6, 2001, http://www.forbes.com/2001/12/06/1206andrx.html.

7. A. Wazana, "Physicians and the Pharmaceutical Industry: Is a Gift Ever Just a Gift?" Journal of the American Medical Association 283 (2000): 373–80. See also Joel Lexchin, "Interactions between Physicians and the Pharmaceutical Industry: What Does the Literature Say?" Canadian Medical Association Journal 149 (1993): 1401–7.

8. Bert Spilker, "The Risks and Benefits of a Pack of M&Ms," Health Affairs 21 (2002): 543–44.

9. James P. Orlowski and Leon Wateska, "The Effects of Pharmaceutical Firm Enticements on Physician Prescribing Patterns: There's No Such Thing as a Free Lunch," Chest 102 (1992): 270–73.

10. Sergio Sismondo, "Pharmaceutical Company Funding and Its Consequences: A Qualitative Systematic Review," Contemporary Clinical Trials 29 (2008): 109–13. See also Joel Lexchin, Lisa Bero, et al., "Pharmaceutical Industry Sponsorship and Research Outcome and Quality: Systematic Review," British Medical Journal 326 (2003): 1167–70.

11. Mary-Margaret Chen and C. Seth Landefeld, "Physicians' Behavior and Their Interactions with Drug Companies: A Controlled Study of Physicians Who Requested Additions to a Hospital Drug Formulary," Journal of the American Medical Association 271 (1994): 684–89.

12. Richard E. Waltman, "I'm at Least as Ethical as a Contractor," Medical Economics 81 (2004): 50–52.

13. Brian Hodge, "Interactions with the Pharmaceutical Industry," Canadian Medical Association Journal 153 (1995): 553–59.

14. M. Asif Ismail, "Drug Lobby Second to None: How the Pharmaceutical Industry Gets Its Way in Washington," Center for Public Integrity Special Report, July 7, 2005, http://projects.publicintegrity.org/rx/report.aspx?aid=723.

15. Public Citizen Congress Watch, "2002 Drug Industry Profits: Hefty Pharmaceutical Company Margins Dwarf Other Industries," June 2003, http://www

.citizen.org/documents/Pharma_Report.pdf. See also Marcia Angell, *The Truth About the Drug Companies* (New York: Random House, 2004), 9.

16. Greg Critser, *Generation Rx* (Boston: Houghton Mifflin, 2005), 100.

17. Robert Steinbrook, "For Sale: Physicians' Prescribing Data," *New England Journal of Medicine* 354 (2006): 2745–47.

18. J. Lee Valentine, "Pharmaceutical Gift Reporting Is an Example of Intolerable Micromanagement," Letters to the Editor, *AMA News*, March 22/29, 2004.

19. Jamie Reidy, *Hard Sell: The Evolution of a Viagra Salesman* (Kansas City, MO: Andrews McMeel Publishing, 2005).

20. Marcel Mauss, *The Gift* (1950; reprint New York: Routledge, 2002), 4.

21. Pierre Bourdieu, *Outline of a Theory of Practice* (Cambridge, UK: Cambridge University Press, 1977). See also Michael Oldani, "Thick Prescriptions: Toward an Interpretation of Pharmaceutical Sales Practices," *Medical Anthropology Quarterly* 18 (2004): 325–56.

22. Frederick S. Sierles, Amy C. Brodkey, et al., "Medical Students' Exposure to and Attitudes About Drug Company Interactions," *Journal of the American Medical Association* 294 (2005): 1034–42.

23. Scott Hensley and Barbara Martinez, "New Treatment: To Sell Their Drugs, Companies Increasingly Rely on Doctors," *Wall Street Journal*, July 15, 2005.

24. John Lantos, *Do We Still Need Doctors?* (New York: Routledge, 1997).

25. Robert Sade, "Medical Care as a Right: A Refutation," *New England Journal of Medicine* 285 (1971): 1288–92.

26. Jeanne Lenzer, "Doctors Refuse Space to Group Fighting Drug Company Influence," *British Medical Journal* 331 (2005): 653.

CHAPTER FOUR: THE THOUGHT LEADERS

1. Donald H. Naftulin, John E. Ware Jr., and Frank A. Donnelly, "The Doctor Fox Lecture: A Paradigm of Educational Seduction," *Journal of Medical Education* 48 (1973): 630–35.

2. Paul Lazarsfeld and Elihu Katz, *Personal Influence: The Part Played by People in the Flow of Mass Communications* (New York: Free Press, 1955).

3. Cutting Edge Information, "Pharmaceutical Thought Leaders: Brand Strategies and Product Positioning," Report PH64 (2004).

4. David C. Radley, Stan N. Finkelstein, and Randall S. Stafford, "Off-Label Prescribing Among Office-Based Physicians," *Archives of Internal Medicine* 166 (2006): 1021–26.

5. Glen Spielmans, "The Promotion of Olanzapine in Primary Care: An Examination of Internal Industry Documents," *Social Science & Medicine* 69 (2009): 14–20. See also Alex Berenson, "Drug Files Show Maker Promoted Unapproved Use," *New York Times*, December 18, 2006, and Gardiner Harris and Alex Berenson, "Settlement Called Near on Zyprexa," *New York Times*, January 15, 2009.

6. Adriane Fugh-Berman and Douglas Melnick, "Off-Label Promotion, On-Target Sales," *PLoS Medicine* 5 (2008): e210. doi:10.1371/journal.pmed.0050210.

7. C. Seth Landefeld and Michael Steinman, "The Neurontin Legacy—Marketing through Misinformation and Manipulation," *New England Journal of Medicine* 360 (2009): 103–6.

8. Jeanne Lenzer, "Pfizer Pleads Guilty, but Drug Sales Continue to Soar," *British Medical Journal* 328 (2004): 1217; and Melody Petersen, "Court Papers Suggest Scale of Drug's Use," *New York Times*, Friday, May 30, 2003.

9. Robert Wilson, *Feminine Forever* (New York: Evans, 1966).

10. Sheila Rothman and David Rothman, *The Pursuit of Perfection: The Promise and Perils of Medical Enhancement* (New York: Pantheon, 2003). The story of Wilson is taken from their account.

11. Alastair Matheson, "Corporate Science and the Husbandry of Scientific and Medical Knowledge by the Pharmaceutical Industry," *Biosocieties* 3 (2008): 355–82.

12. Jacques E. Rossouw, Garnet L. Anderson, Ross L. Prentice, et al., "Risks and Benefits of Estrogen Plus Progestin in Healthy Postmenopausal Women: Principal Results from the Women's Health Initiative Randomized Controlled Trial," *Journal of the American Medical Association* 288 (2002): 321–33.

13. James Samuel Coleman, Elihu Katz, and Herbert Menzel, *Medical Innovation: A Diffusion Study* (Indianapolis: Bobbs-Merrill Co., 1966).

14. Malcolm Gladwell, *The Tipping Point* (Boston: Little, Brown, 2000).

15. Clive Thompson, "Is the Tipping Point Toast?" *Fast Company*, January 28, 2008, http://www.fastcompany.com/magazine/122/is-the-tipping-point-toast .html. See also Duncan Watts, "Challenging the Influentials Hypothesis," in *Measuring Word of Mouth: Current Thinking on Research and Measurement of Word-of-Mouth Marketing* 3, Walter J. Carl, ed. (Chicago: Word of Mouth Marketing Association, 2007), and Duncan Watts, *Six Degrees: The Science of a Connected Age* (New York: W. W. Norton, 2003).

16. Christophe Van den Bulte and Gary L. Lilien, "Medical Innovation Revisited: Social Contagion versus Marketing Effort," *American Journal of Sociology* 106 (2001): 1409–35.

17. Puneet Manchanda, Ying Xie, and Nara Youn, "The Role of Targeted Communication and Contagion in Product Adoption," *Marketing Science* 27 (2008): 961–76.

18. Harikesh Nair, Puneet Manchanda, and Tulikaa Bhatia, "Asymmetric Peer Effects in Physician Prescription Behavior: The Role of Opinion Leaders," Stanford Graduate School of Business Research Paper Series, 2006, http://groups .haas.berkeley.edu/marketing/sics/SICS%202006%20Papers/OPL_June_2006 _V2.pdf.

19. Barry Meier, "2nd Medtronic Consultant Draws Senate's Scrutiny," *New York Times*, July 28, 2009.

20. Christopher Snowbeck, "U Surgeon's Fees Face New Scrutiny—from Payer," *St. Paul Pioneer Press*, July 31, 2009; Janet Moore, "Travel, Meals, All in a $4,000 Day's Work," *Minneapolis Star Tribune*, August 3, 2009. Polly's billing records are included in a letter sent by Senator Grassley to the University of Minnesota, which is posted online at http://stmedia.startribune.com/documents/ polly080209.pdf?elr=KArks:DCiU1OiP:DiiUiacyKUUr.

21. David Armstrong and Thomas M. Burton, "Spine Surgeon Didn't Disclose Medtronic Pay in Testimony," *Wall Street Journal*, July 29, 2009.

22. Gayle White and Craig Schneider, "Emory Psychiatrist as Divisive as He Is Gifted; Dr. Charles B. Nemeroff is a Primary Target of a U.S. Senate Investigation," *Atlanta Journal-Constitution*, October 12, 2008.

23. Shannon Brownlee, "Doctors without Borders," *Washington Monthly*, April 4, 2004, http://www.washingtonmonthly.com/features/2004/0404.brownlee.html.

24. Gardiner Harris, "Leading U.S. Psychiatrist Failed to Report Drug Income," *New York Times*, October 3, 2008.

25. Gardiner Harris, "Drug Maker Told Studies Would Aid It, Papers Say," *New York Times*, March 19, 2009.

26. See Harris, 2009. Biederman's deposition is posted online at http://www.windhover.com/pdf/biedermanday1.pdf and http://www.windhover.com/pdf/biedermanday2.pdf.

27. Sue Pelletier, "Is Pharma Pulling the Strings?" *Medical Meetings* (September/October 2002): 6, http://meetingsnet.com/medicalmeetings/meetings_pharma_pulling_strings/.

28. Sheldon Krimsky, *Science in the Private Interest* (Lanham, MD: Rowman and Littlefield, 2003), 171; Sheldon Krimsky and Les Rothenberg, "Conflict of Interest Policies in Science and Medical Journals: Editorial Practices and Author Disclosures," *Science and Engineering Ethics* 7 (2001): 205–17.

29. Natasha Singer, "Sought-After Speaker, with Script Outlines from Eli Lilly," *New York Times*, November 4, 2009. See also "Lilly's $50,000 Club: The Doctors the Drug Firm Pays the Most," *Pink Sheet*, October 19, 2009.

30. Daylian M. Cain, George Loewenstein, and Don A. Moore, "The Dirt on Coming Clean: Perverse Effects of Disclosing Conflicts of Interest," *Journal of Legal Studies* 34 (2005): 1–25.

31. Jason Dana and George Loewenstein, "A Social Science Perspective on Gifts to Physicians from Industry," *Journal of the American Medical Association* 290 (2003): 252–55.

32. Jeanne Whalen, "Doctor Defends Linking Suicide, Antidepressants," *Wall Street Journal*, July 20, 2004.

33. Peter D. Kramer, *Listening to Prozac: A Psychiatrist Explores Antidepressant Drugs and the Remaking of the Self* (New York: Viking, 1993).

34. Martin Teicher, C. Glod, and J.O. Cole, "Emergence of Intense Suicidal Preoccupation during Fluoxetine Treatment," *American Journal of Psychiatry* 147 (1990): 207–10.

35. David Healy, *The Antidepressant Era* (Cambridge, MA: Harvard University Press, 1997).

36. Mitchell Zuckoff, "Prozac Data Was Kept from Trial, Suit Says," *Boston Globe*, June 8, 2000.

37. R.A. King, M.A. Riddle, P.B. Chappell, et al., "Emergence of Self-Destructive Phenomena in Children and Adolescents during Fluoxetine Treatment," *Journal of the American Academy of Child and Adolescent Psychiatry* 30 (1991): 179–86.

38. John Cornwell, *The Power to Harm* (London: Penguin, 1998).

39. This letter was introduced into evidence during *Fentress v. Eli Lilly*. It is online at http://www.baumhedlundlaw.com/04.pdf.

40. Healy has written about his experience as an expert witness in his book *Let Them Eat Prozac: The Unhealthy Relationship between the Pharmaceutical Industry and Depression* (New York: New York University Press, 2004).

41. Anne McIlroy, "Prozac Critic Sees U of T Job Revoked," *Toronto Globe and*

Mail, April 14, 2001. See also the account on the Canadian Broadcasting Service news documentary program *The National* on July 11, 2001. A detailed chronicle of the CAMH affair was also reported in the *Guardian;* see Sarah Boseley, "Bitter Pill," *Guardian,* May 7, 2001.

42. Karen Birchard, "Scientists Worldwide Protest Withdrawal of Job Offer at U. of Toronto," *Chronicle of Higher Education,* September 11, 2001. See also Owen Dyer, "University Accused of Violating Academic Freedom to Safeguard Funding from Drug Companies," *British Medical Journal* 323 (2001): 591.

43. In that article, I was identified as Healy's "mule" for writing sympathetically about his views.

44. Constance Holden, "Drug Critic Sues after School Pulls Job Offer," *Science* 294 (2001): 29–30. See also Julie Smyth, "Psychiatrist Denied Job Sues U of T: Linked Prozac to Suicide," (Canada) *National Post,* September 25, 2001.

45. Joseph Glenmullen, *Prozac Backlash* (New York: Simon and Schuster, 2000).

46. Sarah Boseley, "'Four People Dead Is Four Too Many,'" *Guardian,* August 9, 2001, http://www.guardian.co.uk/society/2001/aug/09/socialcare.mentalhealth.

47. Jonathan Mahler, "The Antidepressant Dilemma," *New York Times Magazine,* November 21, 2004.

48. Gardiner Harris, "Student, 19, in Trial of New Antidepressant, Commits Suicide," *New York Times,* February 12, 2004; Jeanne Lenzer, "What the FDA Isn't Telling," *Slate,* September 27, 2005, http://www.slate.com/id/2126918/.

49. Sarah Boseley, "Mood Drug Seroxat Banned for Under-18s," *Guardian,* June 11, 2003, http://www.guardian.co.uk/science/2003/jun/11/sciencenews.medicine andhealth.

50. Barbara Martinez, "Glaxo Settles New York Suit over Unpublished Trial Data," *Wall Street Journal,* August 27, 2004, http://online.wsj.com/article/SB109353307148501954.html?mod=googlewsj; BBC News, "Secrets of the Drug Trials," January 29, 2007, http://news.bbc.co.uk/2/hi/programmes/panorama/6291773.stm.

51. Gardiner Harris, "FDA Panel Urges Stronger Warning on Antidepressants," *New York Times,* September 15, 2004, http://query.nytimes.com/gst/fullpage.html ?res=9C05E3DE1E30F936A2575AC0A9629C8B63.

52. Tom Nesi, *Poison Pills: The Untold Story of the Vioxx Drug Scandal* (New York: Thomas Dunne Books, 2008).

53. Milanda Rout, "Vioxx Maker Merck and Co. Drew Up Doctor Hit List," *Australian,* April 1, 2009, http://www.theaustralian.com.au/news/drug-company -drew-up-doctor-hit-list/story-0-1225693586492.

54. Snigdha Prakash, "Documents Suggest Merck Tried to Censor Vioxx Critics," *All Things Considered,* National Public Radio, June 9, 2005; transcripts online at http://www.npr.org/templates/text/s.php?sId=4696609&m=1 and http://www .npr.org/s.php?sId=4696711&m=1.

55. Ibid.

56. Alex Berenson, "Merck Agrees to Settle Vioxx Suits for $4.85 Billion," *New York Times,* November 9, 2007.

57. Liz Kowalczyk, "Perks Policy for Doctors Challenged: Physician Organization Wants Limits Rolled Back," *Boston Globe,* July 23, 2009, http://www.boston

.com/news/local/massachusetts/articles/2009/07/23/new_doctors_group
_challenges_conflict_of_interest_policy_effects/.

58. Daniel Carlat, "Dr. Drug Rep," *New York Times Magazine*, November 25, 2007.

CHAPTER FIVE: THE FLACKS

1. Although I was not asked to keep anything about this meeting confidential, I have refrained from naming the advertising agency, out of courtesy. I have tried to describe the Volkswagen presentation as I remember it. I should also mention that I paid my own expenses for the meeting and did not accept any gifts or an honorarium for my presentation.

2. James Cobb, "2004 Volkswagen Phaeton V-8: A People's Car for Wealthy People," *New York Times*, January 25, 2004.

3. Dan Neil, "Requiem for a Heavyweight," *Los Angeles Times*, April 26, 2006.

4. Al Ries and Laura Ries, *The Fall of Advertising and the Rise of PR* (New York: HarperBusiness, 2002).

5. "Marketing in the Post-Advertising Era": A Panel Discussion at the Harvard Club, New York City, July 11, 2002, http://www.edelman.com/events/Post-Advertising/transcript_w.asp?speed=56.

6. Ries and Ries, *Fall of Advertising*, 90.

7. John Stauber and Sheldon Rampton of the Center for Media and Democracy have been campaigning against VNRs for years. See, for instance, their books *Toxic Sludge Is Good for You! Lies, Damn Lies and the Public Relations Industry* (Monroe, ME: Common Courage Press, 1995) and *Trust Us, We're Experts! How Industry Manipulates Science and Gambles with Your Future* (New York: Jeremy P. Tarcher/Putnam, 2002).

8. Eugene Secunda, "Is TV Addicted to Drug Company PR?" *Business and Society Review* 73 (1990): 11–13.

9. The Center for Media and Democracy published a comprehensive report on VNRs in 2006. See Diane Farsetta and Daniel Price, "Fake TV News: Widespread and Undisclosed," Center for Media and Democracy, April 6, 2006, http://www.prwatch.org/fakenews/execsummary.

10. "'Press' Love Affair with Viagra Is a Powerful PR Potion," *PR News* 54 (1998): 19.

11. http://www.thepsaexperts.com/.

12. http://www.thepsaexperts.com/getting_psas.html (accessed May 19, 2009).

13. Stuart Ewen, *PR! A Social History of Spin* (New York: Basic Books, 1996), 159–62.

14. Ibid, 161.

15. Larry Tye, *The Father of Spin: Edward L. Bernays and the Birth of Public Relations* (New York: Henry Holt, 2002).

16. Edward L. Bernays, "The Engineering of Consent," *Annals of the American Academy of Political and Social Science* 250 (1947): 113–20.

17. Tye, *Father of Spin*, 28–30.

18. Ewen, *PR!* 167.

19. Edward L. Bernays, *Propaganda* (1928; reprint New York: Ig Publishing,

2005), 71. The full text of *Propaganda* is available online at http://www.archive.org/details/Propaganda_600.

20. Ewen, *PR!* 166.

21. Mark Crispin Miller makes this point in his excellent introduction to the 2005 edition of *Propaganda*.

22. Bernays, *Propaganda*, 38.

23. Ibid., 78.

24. David Healy, *The Antidepressant Era* (Cambridge, MA: Harvard University Press, 1997), 83.

25. Reinhard Angelmar, Sarah Angelmar, and Liz Kane, "Building Strong Condition Brands," *Journal of Medical Marketing* 7 (2007): 341–51. Critics call this *disease-mongering*, a term that is often attributed to Lynn Payer. See Lynn Payer, *Disease-Mongers* (New York: Wiley, 1994).

26. Vince Parry, "Disease Branding: What Is It, Why It Works, and How to Do It," *Pharmaceutical Executive*, supplement (2007): 22–24.

27. Steven Woloshin and Lisa Schwartz, "Giving Legs to Restless Legs: A Case Study of How the Media Helps Make People Sick," *PLoS Medicine* 3 (2006): e170 .doi:10.1371/journal.pmed.0030170.

28. "FTC Clears Way for Pfizer Acquisition of Pharmacia," Associated Press, *USA Today*, April 14, 2003, http://www.usatoday.com/money/industries/health/drugs/2003-04-14-pfizer-pharmacia_x.htm.

29. Angelmar, Angelmar, and Kane, "Building Strong."

30. Joseph Davis, "Adolescents and the Pathologies of the Achieving Self," *Hedgehog Review* 11 (2009): 37–49.

31. Ian Hacking, "Making Up People," *London Review of Books* 28 (2006): 23–26.

32. A lively account of the changes leading up to direct-to-consumer advertising of prescription drugs can be found in Greg Critser, *Generation Rx* (Boston: Houghton Mifflin, 2005).

33. Thomas J. Lueck, "At Lilly, the Side Effects of Oraflex," *New York Times*, August 15, 1982, http://www.nytimes.com/1982/08/15/business/at-lilly-the-side-effects-of-oraflex.html?&pagewanted=all. See also Critser, *Generation Rx*, 32–34.

34. Jeremy Greene, *Prescribing by Numbers: Drugs and the Definition of Disease* (Baltimore: Johns Hopkins University Press, 2007), 38.

35. Critser, *Generation Rx*, 36.

36. Henry J. Kaiser Family Foundation, "The Impact of Direct to Consumer Advertising on Prescription Drug Spending," Menlo Park, CA, 2003, http://www.kff.org/rxdrugs/loader.cfm?url=/commonspot/security/getfile.cfm&PageID=14378.

37. Julie M. Donohue, Marisa Cevasco, and Meredith B. Rosenthal, "A Decade of Direct-to-Consumer Advertising of Prescription Drugs," *New England Journal of Medicine* 357 (2007): 673–81.

38. http://www.pharmalot.com/2008/09/merck-vioxx-cox-in-paradise-tom-nesi-explains/.

39. Gina Kolata, "Merck and Vioxx: The Overview," *New York Times*, October 1, 2004, http://query.nytimes.com/gst/fullpage.html?res=940CE3DD1338F932A357 53C1A9629C8B63&sec=&spon=&pagewanted=all.

40. Stephanie Saul, "Fen-Phen Case Lawyers Say They'll Reject Wyeth Offer,"

New York Times, February 17, 2005, http://query.nytimes.com/gst/fullpage.html ?res=9505E7D6133AF934A25751C0A9639C8B63.

41. Darren Rovell, "The Burden of Pitching Pills," ESPN.com, November 19, 2004, http://sports.espn.go.com/espn/print?id=1927023&type=story. See also Eric J. Topol, "Failing the Public Health: Rofecoxib, Merck, and the FDA," *New England Journal of Medicine* 351 (2004): 1707–9.

42. Associated Press, "Merck Agrees to Settlement over Vioxx Ads," May 21, 2008, http://www.nytimes.com/2008/05/21/business/21vioxx.html.

43. John Simons, "Blockbusters to the Rescue," *Fortune*, January 31, 2006, http://money.cnn.com/magazines/fortune/fortune_archive/2006/01/23/8366988/index.htm.

44. Bernays, *Propaganda*, 76. See also "Freud's Nephew and the Origins of Public Relations," National Public Radio, http://www.npr.org/templates/story/story.php?storyId=4612464.

45. Critser, *Generation Rx*, 26.

46. Bob Burton and Andy Rowell, "From Patient Activism to Astroturf Marketing," *PR Watch* 10 (2003), http://www.prwatch.org/prwissues/2003Q1/astroturf .html.

47. Melissa Healy, "Selling the Patient," *Los Angeles Times*, August 6, 2007. See also Jessica Marshall and Peter Aldhous, "Patient Groups Special: Swallowing the Best Advice?" *New Scientist*, October 27, 2006, http://www.newscientist.com/article/mg19225755.100.

48. Gardiner Harris, "Drug Makers Are Advocacy Group's Biggest Donors," *New York Times*, October 21, 2009.

49. Ken Silverstein, "Prozac.org," *Mother Jones*, November/December 1999, http://motherjones.com/politics/1999/11/prozacorg.

50. Gina Kolata, "Selling Growth Drug for Children: The Legal and Ethical Questions," *New York Times*, August 15, 1994, http://www.nytimes.com/1994/08/15/us/selling-growth-drug-for-children-the-legal-and-ethical-questions .html?pagewanted=all.

51. Ralph King, "Charity Tactic by Genentech Stirs Questions," *Wall Street Journal*, August 10, 1994.

52. "Alzheimer's Campaign Peaks Public and Media Interest," *PR News* 57 (2001).

53. Ray Moynihan and Alan Cassels, *Selling Sickness* (New York: Nation Books, 2005), 42.

54. See the "Celebrity Causes and Disease Awareness Campaign" section of the Brooks International speakers' bureau Web site at http://www.brooksinternational.com/RelId/605904/ISvars/default/Celebrity_Causes_%2526_Disease _Awareness_Campaigns.htm.

55. Shirley S. Wang, "A Celebrity Patient's Backing Turns Sour for Drug Company," *Wall Street Journal*, May 14, 2009.

56. "Big Pharma, Big Phiction," *On the Media*, National Public Radio, October 21, 2005; transcript at http://www.onthemedia.org/yore/transcripts/transcripts _102105_pharma.html.

57. Shannon Brownlee and Jeanne Lenzer, "Truth Is Stranger Than Phiction," *Slate*, November 29, 2005, http://www.slate.com/id/2131200/.

CHAPTER SIX: THE ETHICISTS

1. Antonio Regalado, "*To Sell Pricey Drug, Eli Lilly Fuels a Debate over Rationing,*" *Wall Street Journal*, September 18, 2003. See also Carl Elliott, "Not So Public Relations," *Slate*, December 15, 2003, http://www.slate.com/id/2092442/; and Peter Q. Eichacker, Charles Natanson, and Robert L. Danner, "Surviving Sepsis—Practice Guidelines, Marketing Campaigns, and Eli Lilly," *New England Journal of Medicine* 355 (2006): 1640–42.

2. Laurie Zoloth, "Heroic Measures: Just Bioethics in an Unjust World," *Hastings Center Report* 31 (2001): 34–40.

3. Council of Public Relations, "Eli Lilly, Belsito, Surviving Sepsis: Case Studies—Marketing Communications of Public Relations," http://www.prfirms.org/resources/case_studies/Marketing_Communications/2004/SurvivingSepsis1.asp.

4. The funding of the Ethics Resource Center changes over time, but a current list of funders is disclosed on its Web site at http://www.ethics.org/about-erc/donors-sponsors. Its annual reports have additional information at http://www.ethics.org/page/how-we-are-funded.

5. Harold Shapiro's CV is online at Princeton University at http://www.princeton.edu/ffihts/PDFs/Shapiro_CV.pdf.

6. Adam Sichko, "In Transition, McGee Turns to Growing a Bioethics Business for Profit," *Business Review* (Albany), August 29, 2008, http://albany.bizjournals.com/albany/stories/2008/09/01/story6.html?b=1220241600^1692509.

7. See http://www.e-four.org/Home/about-crucial-choices.

8. See Weinstein's Web page at http://www.theethicsguy.com.

9. Carl Elliott, "Pharma Buys a Conscience," *American Prospect* 12 (2001): 16–20; Sheryl Stolberg, "Bioethicists Fall Under Familiar Scrutiny," *New York Times*, August 2, 2001.

10. Stolberg, "Bioethicists Fall."

11. For Moreno, see his Web page at the University of Pennsylvania: http://hss.sas.upenn.edu/mt-static/faculty/department_faculty/jonathan_moreno_phd_professor.php. For Beauchamp and Levine, see the Eli Lilly Corporate Citizenship Report 2005–06, online at http://www.socialfunds.com/csr/reports/Lilly_2005–2006_Corporate_Citizenship_Report.pdf. For Childress, see the University of Virginia Center for Bioethics Ethics Annual Report, 2002–03.

12. Baruch Brody, Nancy Dubler, et al., "Bioethics Consultation in the Private Sector," *Hastings Center Report* 32 (2002): 14–20, http://repository.upenn.edu/cgi/viewcontent.cgi?article=1024&context=bioethics_papers.

13. Thomas Donaldson, "The Business Ethics of Bioethics Consulting," *Hastings Center Report* 31 (2001): 12–14.

14. Stephen Hall, *Merchants of Immortality: Chasing the Dream of Human Life Extension* (Boston: Houghton Mifflin, 2003), 321, 323.

15. Laurie P. Cohen, "Stuck for Money," *Wall Street Journal*, November 14, 1996.

16. Tom Beauchamp, Bruce Jennings, Eleanor Kinney, and Robert Levine, "Pharmaceutical Research Involving the Homeless," *Journal of Medicine and Philosophy* 27 (2002): 547–64.

17. Stolberg, "Bioethicists Fall."

18. Maurice Pappworth, *Human Guinea Pigs* (Boston: Beacon Press, 1967).

19. Sandra Coney and Phillida Bunkle, "An 'Unfortunate Experiment' at National Women's," *Metro* (1987): 47–65; Alastair V. Campbell, "A Report from New Zealand: An 'Unfortunate Experiment,' " *Bioethics* 3 (1989): 59–66.

20. David Rothman, "Were Tuskegee and Willowbrook 'Studies in Nature'?" *Hastings Center Report* (1982): 5–7; James Jones, *Bad Blood: The Tuskegee Syphilis Experiment* (New York: Free Press, 1981).

21. Shana Alexander, "They Decide Who Lives, Who Dies," *Life* 53 (1962): 102–25.

22. Albert Jonsen, *The Birth of Bioethics* (New York: Oxford University Press, 1998), 212.

23. Mark Siegler, "Ethics Committees: Decisions by Bureaucracy," *Hastings Center Report* 16 (1986): 22–24; Mark Siegler and Peter Singer, "Clinical Ethics Consultation: Godsend or 'God Squad'?" *American Journal of Medicine* 85 (1988): 759–60.

24. Eils Lotozo, "Bioethicist Foresees a Wild Frontier in Genetics Field," *Philadelphia Inquirer*, October 28, 2003.

25. Glenn McGee, *Beyond Genetics* (New York: HarperCollins, 2003), 6.

26. James Hughes, *Citizen Cyborg* (New York: Westview Press, 2004), 21, 92.

27. Jonathan Imber, "Medical Publicity before Bioethics: Nineteenth-Century Illustrations of Twentieth-Century Dilemmas," in Raymond DeVries and Janardan Subedi (eds.), *Bioethics and Society: Constructing the Ethical Enterprise* (New York: Prentice Hall, 1998), 30.

28. Sheryl Gay Stolberg, "FDA Officials Fault Penn Team in Gene Therapy Death," *New York Times*, December 9, 1999; online at http://partners.nytimes .com/library/national/science/health/120999hth-gene-therapy.html.

29. Joanne Silberner, "A Gene Therapy Death," *Hastings Center Report* 30 (2000): 118; Trudo Lemmens, "Confronting the Conflict of Interest Crisis in Medical Research," *Monash Bioethics Review* 23 (2004): 19–40.

30. Arthur Caplan and David Magnus, "Overregulating Research," *Chicago Tribune*, December 21, 1999.

31. Benjamin Freedman, "Where Are the Heroes of Bioethics?" *Journal of Clinical Ethics* 7 (1996): 297–99.

32. The Pfizer press release is online at http://www.pfizerhumanhealth.co.za/ runtime/popcontentrun.aspx?pageidref=2226.

33. "Grant from Pfizer Foundation Allows Establishment of Centre for Medical Humanities at UCL," *Journal of Medical Ethics: Medical Humanities* 27 (2001): 69.

34. The Center for Practical Bioethics has posted a list of contributors at http://www.practicalbioethics.org/FileUploads/Contributions%20to%20the %20Center.May%202008.pdf.

35. "Merck Visiting Scholars," *Seton Hall Law* 6 (2004): 23, online at http://law .shu.edu/publications/Alumni/upload/vol6_issue2.pdf. The Center for Health and Pharmaceutical Law and Policy discloses its funding online at http://law .shu.edu/ProgramsCenters/HealthTechIP/Disclosure-Statement.cfm.

36. A press release is available at http://law.wlu.edu/news/storydetail.asp ?id=516.

37. *Hastings Center Activities Report* 2007–08, online at http://www.the

hastingscenter.org/uploadedFiles/Support_Us/07–08%20activities%20report
.pdf.

38. http://www.giving.utoronto.ca/chairs/showchairs.asp?ID=135.

39. Carl Elliott, "Throwing a Bone to the Watchdog," *Hastings Center Report*
31 (2001): 9–12.

40. U.S. Government Accountability Office, "Human Subjects Research:
Undercover Tests Show the Institutional Review Board System Is Vulnerable to
Unethical Manipulation" (Washington, DC: U.S. Government Accountability Office, 2009), http://www.gao.gov/new.items/d09448t.pdf.

41. Alicia Mundy, "Sting Operation Exposes Gaps in Oversight of Human Experiments," *Wall Street Journal*, March 26, 2009; "Congress Vents Outrage at FDA,
OHRP and IRBs," *Clinical Trials Advisor* 14 (2009).

42. The commercial has been posted on YouTube at http://www.youtube
.com/watch?v=6FnpRihIUH8.

43. Barry Meier, "An Overseer of Trials Draws Fire," *New York Times*, March
26, 2009.

44. The hearings on the results of the sting operation were conducted by the
House Energy and Commerce Committee's Subcommittee on Oversight and Investigations on March 26, 2009. The transcript is posted online at http://energy
commerce.house.gov/Press_111/20090326/transcript_20090326_oi.pdf. Videos of
the hearing are also posted there.

45. Dueber's testimony is posted on the Energy and Commerce Committee
Web site at http://energycommerce.house.gov/Press_111/20090326/testimony
_dueber.pdf.

46. See page 77 of the transcript of the hearing.

47. Jill Fisher, *Medical Research for Hire: The Political Economy of Pharmaceutical Clinical Trials* (Piscataway, NJ: Rutgers University Press, 2008), 11.

48. Heidi Ledford, "Trial and Error," *Nature* 448 (2007): 530–32.

49. The funding problem for commercial IRBs mirrors the problem for the
FDA that was introduced by the widely criticized Prescription Drug User Fee Act
(PDUFA), which authorized the FDA to collect user fees from drug companies that
produce certain products. When the PDUFA was enacted in 1992, it was intended
to speed up drug approvals, mainly by funding additional employees. In practice, it has made the FDA financially dependent on the pharmaceutical industry,
much like commercial IRBs are. "PDUFA transformed the way the FDA operates,"
says Erick Turner, a former FDA drug reviewer who is now on the faculty at Oregon Health Science Center. PDUFA mandated strict timelines for drug approvals and periodic meetings between industry and FDA officials. "So the industry
bought access to the FDA—basically, now they get to be in their face constantly,"
says Turner. "Now the FDA seems to view industry as its primary client, with an
approved drug being the product of that relationship." But in the decade after
PDUFA was introduced, an unprecedented thirteen drugs had to be withdrawn
from the market after proving to be dangerous. See Marcia Angell, *The Truth
About the Drug Companies* (New York: Random House, 2003).

50. http://www.goodwynirb.com/Home.htm.

51. The transcripts of the presentation are online at http://www.bioethics
.gov/transcripts/sep02/session2.html.

52. Alicia Mundy, "Was a Three-Legged Dog Head of a Review Board?" *Wall*

Street Journal Health Blog, March 26, 2009, http://blogs.wsj.com/health/2009/03/26/was-a-three-legged-dog-head-of-a-review-board/.

53. Fredric L. Coe, "The Costs and Benefits of a Well-Intended Parasite: A Witness and Reporter on the IRB Phenomenon," *Northwestern University Law Review* 101 (2007): 723–33.

54. E. G. Campbell et al., "Characteristics of Medical School Faculty Members Serving on Institutional Review Boards: Results of a National Survey," *Academic Medicine* 78 (2004): 769–74. See also Christine Vogeli, Greg Koski, and Eric Campbell, "Policies and Management of Conflicts of Interest within Medical Research Institutional Review Boards: Results of a National Study," *Academic Medicine* 84 (2009): 488–94.

55. Jeremy Sugarman, Kenneth Getz, et al., "The Cost of Institutional Review Boards in Academic Health Centers," *New England Journal of Medicine* 352 (2005): 1825–27.

56. http://cflegacy.research.umn.edu/irb/bandi.cfm.

57. See the news archives on the Western IRB Web site at http://www.wirb.com/content/foot_wirb_news_archive.aspx.

58. Adil Shamoo and Elizabeth Woeckner, "Research Ethics Boards: No Data on Quality of For-Profit or Non-Profit IRBs," *PLoS Medicine* 3 (2006): e459. Online at http://www.plosmedicine.org/article/info:doi/10.1371/journal.pmed.0030459.

59. Robert Whitaker, "Lure of Riches Fuels Testing," *Boston Globe*, November 17, 1998.

60. David Evans, Michael Smith, and Liz Willen, "Private Tests a Risky Business," *Seattle Times*, November 7, 2005.

61. Liz Willen and David Evans, "Artist Grows Increasingly Ill in Test," *Seattle Times*, November 7, 2005.

62. "Western IRB Sells Majority Stake to Boston Ventures," *CW Weekly* 11 (2007): 1, 3.

63. Eric Engleman, "Research-Review Company Emerges as a Pivotal Player," *Puget Sound Business Journal*, March 30, 2007, http://seattle.bizjournals.com/seattle/stories/2007/04/02/story2.html.

64. The video, called "The Viagra Case Study," is online at http://www.washingtonspeakers.com/scripts/flvplayer/flvplayer.cfm?src=art_caplan_d_viagra_case_study.

65. Janet Moore, "U Medical School Plan: Ban All Gifts to Doctors," *Minneapolis Star Tribune*, October 21, 2008.

66. Reed Abelson, "Whistle-Blower Suit Says Device Maker Generously Rewards Doctors," *New York Times*, January 24, 2006.

67. http://www.harrisinteractive.com/harris_poll/index.asp?PID=611. See also Margaret Eaton, "Managing the Risks Associated with Using Biomedical Ethics Advice," *Journal of Business Ethics* 77 (2008): 99–109.

INDEX

AAFP. *See* American Academy of Family Physicians (AAFP)

Abilify, 133–34

Abuzzahab, Faruk, 8–10

academic health centers: and bioethicists, 148, 150, 157; drug studies in, 2–3, 9, 11; financial needs of, 84; and institutional review boards (IRBs), 162–63; and medical care for injured drug research subjects, 21; slow pace of drug studies in, 3. *See also* physician-researchers

academic physicians. *See* physician-researchers

ACCME. *See* Accreditation Council for Continuing Medical Education (ACCME)

Accreditation Council for Continuing Medical Education (ACCME), 28

ACE inhibitors, 136

ACNP. *See* American College of Neuropsychopharmacology (ACNP)

ACRE. *See* Association of Clinical Researchers and Educators (ACRE)

activism by/for guinea pigs, 18–21

ACT UP, 129

Adams, Phyllis, 63

ADHD. *See* attention deficit hyperactivity disorder (ADHD)

Advanced Cell Technology, 143, 144–45

advertising: blockbuster model of, 127–28; consumer (DTC) advertising, xiii, 52, 54, 60, 115, 124–28; cost of television ads, 115; culture of, and medical communication, 38–39, 47–48; estrogen replacement ad campaign, 82; marketing and public relations versus, 111–12; in medical journals, 39, 41, 52, 124, 125; by physicians, 53; return on investment for, 52, 126; Roselin's criticisms of, 134–37; Volkswagen campaign, 109–11. *See also* marketing of drugs

advocacy by/for guinea pigs, 18–21

African Americans, 4, 5, 147

Agriculture Department, Bureau of Chemistry, 16

AIDS, 60, 129–30

akathisia, 98–99

Albany Medical School, 142

Alda, Alan, 132

Alexander, Shana, 147

Allergan, 112

Alzheimer's Association, 132, 133

Alzheimer's disease, 7, 115, 132–33

AMA. *See* American Medical Association (AMA)

Amazon.com, 111

American Academy of Family Physicians (AAFP), 45, 72

journals published for, 41–42; and
publication planning, 28–31; and
public relations, 111, 119–22; and
review articles, 36–37; Roselin's
criticisms of, 134–37; scandals
in, 42–47; size and scope of, 42,
45–47; and thalidomide, 42–44; and
third-party technique, 128–34; and
thought leaders, 75–108; and Viagra,
169. *See also* advertising; drug reps;
medical communication; public
relations; thought leaders
Massachusetts General Hospital, 91
Massachusetts Medical Society, 46
Matheson, Alastair, 82
Mauss, Marcel, 64
Mayo Clinic, 84
McCormick, Richard, 148
McGee, Glenn, 142, 151
McGill University, 153, 162–63, 168
McKinney, Dwight, 145
MECC (medical education and
communications companies), 27
med-check clinics, 72–73
med comms, 27. *See also* medical
communication
med ed companies, 27. *See also* medical
education
medical communication: and
advertising agency culture, 38–39,
47–48; Bronstein on, 25–26, 29,
34, 35–36, 38–39, 49; and decision
to spin or bury data, 35–36; and
ethical problems with ghostwriting,
31–34, 47–48; on Fen-Phen, 44–46;
Gilbert on, 31, 38, 39; Logdberg
on, 35, 37–38, 47–48; mechanics
of ghostwriting, 29; and medical
education, 27–28, 45–47, 57–58; and
medical journals, 29–30, 39–42, 45;
pseudo-medical journals published
for drug marketing, 41–42; and
publication planning, 28–31; and
reprint articles from medical
journals, 41; review articles as,
36–37; statistics on ghostwriting
of, 29–31; statistics on U.S. med
comms, 27; tension between

science and commerce in, 34–39;
on thalidomide, 42–44; by thought
leaders, 78–81; types of, 36–37. *See
also* ghostwriting
medical education, 27–28, 45–47,
57–58. *See also* Continuing Medical
Education (CME)
medical ghostwriting. *See* ghostwriting
Medical Innovation (Katz, Coleman,
and Menzel), 85–88
medical journals, 29–30, 39–42, 45, 52,
124, 125. *See also specific journals*
Medical Letter, 53
Medical Meetings, 92
medical research. *See* drug studies
Medical Review of Reviews, 117
medical students, 56, 68–69, 72
Medical University of South Carolina, 71
medical writers. *See* ghostwriting
Medicare, 130
medicine: changes in, xiv–xv, 46–47,
71–72; corporate-style medicine, 53–
56, 72; deception in, ix–xi; Internet
changes compared with, xiv–xv;
pharmaceutical industry's impact
on, xi–xiv, 72, 102; professional
ethics code for, xv; status in medical
world, 84. *See also* pharmaceutical
industry; physicians
Medtronic, 88–89
meningitis, 10–11
menopause, 81–84
Menrium, 82
mental illness. *See* antipsychotic drugs;
psychiatric clinical trials; psychiatry
and psychiatrists; schizophrenia;
suicide and suicidal ideation
Menzel, Herbert, 85–88
Merchants of Immortality (Hall), 144
Merck: and AIDS activists, 130; and
antidepressants, 120; discrediting
of dissenting thought leaders by,
103–5; drug reps for, 53–54, 59; and
drug research subjects, 7; funding of
bioethics organizations by, 153–56;
gifts from drug reps of, xii; lawsuits
against, 104, 127; public image of,
127; and Singulair, 114; thought

ABOUT THE AUTHOR

CARL ELLIOTT teaches at the Center for Bioethics at the University of Minnesota. A graduate of Davidson College, Elliott earned his MD at the Medical University of South Carolina and a PhD in philosophy at Glasgow University in Scotland. He has taught at universities in Canada, South Africa, and New Zealand. In 2003–04, he was visiting associate professor at the Institute for Advanced Study in Princeton, New Jersey.

Elliott is the author or editor of six previous books, including *Better Than Well: American Medicine Meets the American Dream*. His articles have appeared in the *New Yorker* and *Atlantic Monthly* as well as the *New England Journal of Medicine*. A native South Carolinian, Elliott lives in Minneapolis with his wife, Ina, and his three children, Crawford, Martha, and Lyle.